705.4 ✓

D0118552

Catch a Falling Star

Catch a Falling Star
Living with Alzheimer's

by
Betty Baker Spohr
with
Jean Valens Bullard

STORM PEAK PRESS

SEATTLE, WASHINGTON

To The Man I Married

STORM PEAK PRESS

157 YESLER WAY, SUITE 413

SEATTLE, WASHINGTON 98104

© Copyright 1995, Betty Baker Spohr and Jean Valens Bullard
ISBN 0-9641357-1-X
Library of Congress Catalog Card Number: 95-15655

Library of Congress Cataloging-in-Publication Data
Spohr, Betty Baker.
    Catch a falling star : living with Alzheimer's / by Betty
    Baker Spohr, with Jean Valens Bullard : foreword by Roger
    B. Hickler.
            p.   cm.
        ISBN 0-9641357-1-X
        1. Alzheimer's disease--Patients--Biography.
    2. Alzheimer's disease--Patients--Family relationships.
    3. Spohr, Betty Baker--Family. I. Bullard, Jean Valens.
    II. Title.
    RC523.2.S66 1995
    362.1'96831--dc20   95-15655

Go and catch a falling star . . .
Tell me where all past years are
　　　— John Donne (circa 1596)

Foreword

The author has produced a remarkable picture-story of her personal experience with Alzheimer's disease. It is a moving account of her home supervision over the ten-year period when her husband, a devoted partner, passes through the increasingly severe phases of this inexorable disorder. Through the author-artist's eyes we see an accomplished energetic engineer gradually decline into a disordered being requiring constant attention.

Physicians may describe these cumulative mental and physical losses, due to progressive neuronal wasting, in precise technical terms. They will not do as well as Betty Spohr in conveying either the clinical phenomena or the personal impact. To have undertaken this task is commendable. To have done it with such wit, honesty and intelligence is prodigious.

Advances of medical science have afforded greater longevity, and an unwanted by-product is the increasing incidence of Alzheimer's disease. There are now few multi-generational families that have not borne some of the burden, and this highly readable book will give real comfort to many in similar circumstances.

For readers in general, it is a stirring confirmation of the best that is in the human spirit. The poignant illustrations contribute as much to the story as the prose.

Roger B. Hickler, M. D.
Lamar Soutter Distinguished Professor of Medicine, Emeritus
University of Massachusetts Medical Center
Worcester, Massachusetts

Preface

The man I loved and married slowly disappeared as Alzheimer's disease inevitably took its toll. It was painful to look at him and remember the always-in-a-hurry Hank running up every flight of stairs two or three steps at a time. I'd imagine him active and energetic and in complete control of himself, his life, his job. I'd see him as an operations engineer supervising a staff of several hundred. I'd picture him, so pleased with himself yet trying not to show it, when he'd been able to help some hard-working but struggling employee realize his or her full potential. The long- and short-range plans he made for his job and his family never failed to work out for everyone's benefit. Never demonstrative, he would show his love shyly with a bunch of long-stemmed red roses and a white one for each of our three children. Alzheimer's disease relentlessly took that Hank away from me.

Along the way I was besieged by all kinds of unwanted feelings: resentment that this dire thing should attack Hank just when, after having spent twenty-five years working in Asia and Africa, he was going to have a chance to do all the things he'd dreamed of doing during his retirement; self-pity as I began to have less and less freedom; guilt, fearing I was not doing enough, or the right things for him; embarrassment when he exhibited erratic, strange behavior; anger and impatience when he became impossibly stubborn about something I felt should be done immediately.

As it was so devastating to compare this progressively incapable man with the forceful, dynamic man in my memory, I tried, though not always successfully, to develop an impersonal approach to my caregiving. To get me through I tried to forget Hank as my husband and thought of him as a patient to be carefully tended.

I'm not quite sure why I started to "draw" Hank's illness. I may have thought a record of his progress and/or decline would be helpful. Surprisingly enough, it also turned out to be therapy for me.

As my freedoms became more and more restricted, I needed something to occupy my mind and hands. When I'm not busy doing something of my own, I feel useless and depressed. It would seem that to submerge myself in the very thing that was causing my confinement would only add to the problem. It worked in just the opposite way.

In trying to chronicle the events as they occurred and to depict them in a humane way, I began to look for the humorous things, and there were many. Recording it all helped me to clarify information and find possible solutions.

I realize, of course, that every AD case differs from every other, that time and event sequences and disease duration vary. Still, as my "picture story" progressed, I began to think that, though this was my own personal experience, what I was going through might in some ways be similar to what so many people face, or might face down the road. Perhaps others, looking through it, might be helped to anticipate a few of the hazards and be prepared (if one ever can be) for things to come. Perhaps

it would point up some of the seemingly unanswerable
questions: what to do about doctors, lawyers, business
affairs; when and where to get help? I don't pretend to
know more than a portion of the answers, and I never
will know the rest, but posing the questions may help
others to know some of the difficulties and help them
plan appropriate action before crises occur.

Florence Powers, the wife of a good friend of Hank's,
was diagnosed as having Alzheimer's disease some years
before Hank. For six summers, Florence and Ed came to
visit us. During those years Florence, whom we never
knew as a well woman, went from being lucid but
faltering, to wholly incoherent and shuffling. It was soon
after these summer visits began that I knew Hank was in
the beginning stages of the same disease. Since we saw
Florence only once a year, the changes were dramatic,
and often devastating.

Ed, a busy contractor, cared for Florence at home,
with minimal help, for over ten years. Finally, violence
and resistance made it impossible. About six months
after their last visit Florence died in a nursing home.

Talking with Ed alone, watching and talking with
Florence and Ed together, helped me to anticipate many
of the pitfalls, and have some idea of what was in store
for me. Changes in Hank weren't easy, but most were
expected, and therefore less traumatic.

When Ed read this picture-story, I told him how much
my observing Florence and his care of her had helped me
anticipate and cope. Ed said, "That's what your book can
do for others." I hope so.

Betty Baker Spohr

Catch a Falling Star

Hovering there, it seems so close
an outstretched hand could brush
its fragile tip.
When I reach to touch
it shies away to settle furtively
upon a nearby hill.
Like some wild scavenger
it waits in readiness to flee,
yet wanting desperately to stay.
Approaching softly,
pausing now and then
to let a bit of star-shine
soothe my face,
I come within a needle's space.
Clouds mist out that lovely light.
Darkness comes.

I

The Verdict . . .
Everything Changes

THE FIRST FIVE YEARS

First Year Spring, Cape Cod

Hank's first year of retirement: we've just returned to our Cape Cod, Massachusetts, home after living for twenty-five years in the tropics.

During his first annual physical checkup after retiring, Hank asks why his memory isn't as good as it used to be. Almost total recall is something on which he has always prided himself.

After a series of exhaustive tests and after ruling out all other possibilities, the doctor tells me:

Hank must have ALZHEIMER'S!

The doctor's explanation leaves me in shock. There's no cure. There's no really effective medical help available. It's downhill all the way.

Alzheimer's disease (AD) is something about which I know almost nothing. What will this mean to Hank? To me?

Whether or not to tell Hank what's the matter is a difficult decision. The doctor leaves it up to me. An incurable optimist and fighter, how would Hank cope with knowing what is in store for him? If he guesses and asks me directly, how will I tell him?

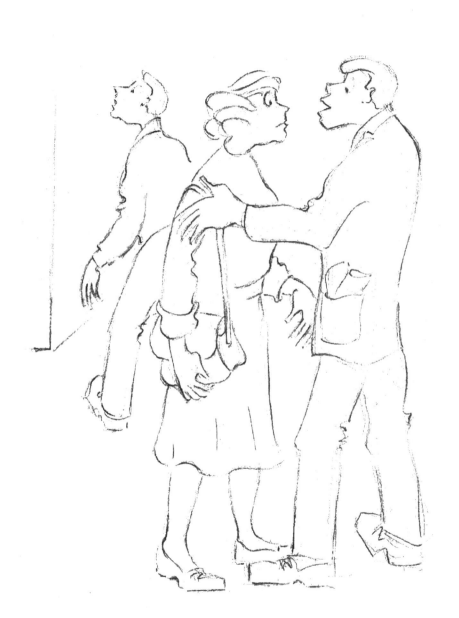

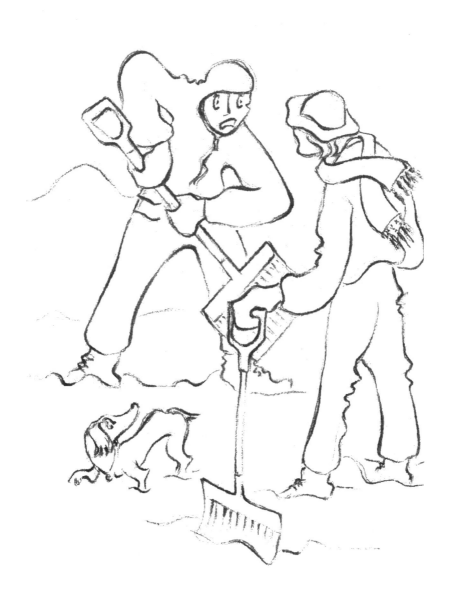

First Year Winter, Cape Cod

In spite of what I have just learned, with no first-hand experience of what lies ahead, I want to ignore the whole problem.

We spend a few glorious days in REAL Vermont snow: cross-country skiing, tramping the woods.

But . . . we arrive at Cape Cod at three P.M. to find five inches of the white stuff covering our driveway. It has to be cleared before dark.

Hank, at five-foot-seven-inches, tops me by four inches, but unlike me, he hasn't an ounce of fat on him. He shivers as the temperature drops, and gets more unhappy with each shovelful. He swears NEVER to do this again!

Second Year Spring, Cape Cod

Our friends Ed and Florence Powers come for a visit. Florence has had Alzheimer's for some time. It was finally diagnosed after several futile years searching for the cause of her growing disabilities.

She's already quite limited, but can still communicate rather haltingly. She knows what the future will bring. All of us talk about it openly.

Hank is kind, helpful and concerned for her. He never even intimates that he thinks his memory loss might be due to Alzheimer's, too. I can't believe he hasn't guessed. He *must* be denying this to himself. I'll never tell him now.

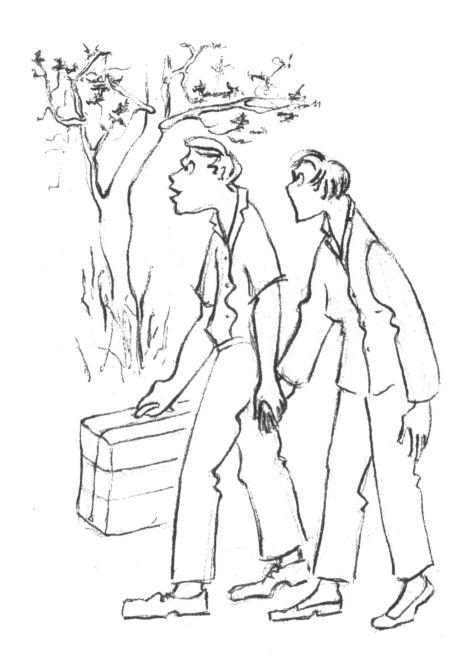

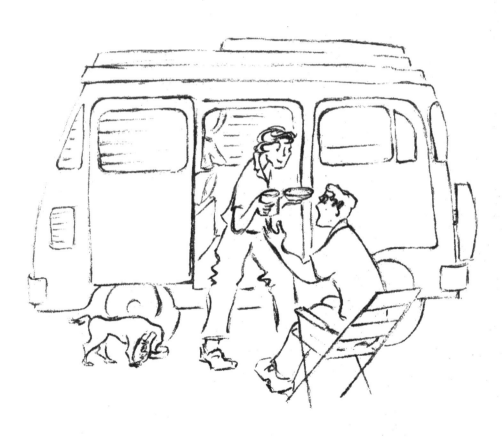

Second Year Summer, Traveling

Our life feels so normal, I get excited when Hank decides what we need is a camper. He comes up with a vivid yellow VW pop-top.

Hank's aim: to get out of New England's winter cold and into someplace warm. Our lively French poodle, Noni (whose name means young lady in Malay), agrees.

We make an exploratory run down the east coast, across Florida's panhandle, through the Gulf states, and then head for California.

On our way we check out Sun City West, Arizona. Both in our sixties, we qualify for a retirement community. Do we want it? Is this the "warm place" for us?

A month later, we take the plunge, sign on the dotted line for a house in Sun City West, then go back to Cape Cod to wait for our Arizona house to be built and ready for occupancy.

On the way to Cape Cod, we start making plans for furnishing our new western home and dream of the "good life" we'll live each winter in warm (we hope) Arizona.

Third Year Winter, Cape Cod

I go on a picture-hanging binge. When I ask Hank for a hammer, he goes off merrily in search of one . . . to the fridge!

At first I'm annoyed. Hank usually seems so "normal." *Why is he so stupid? How could I have married anyone so dense?* These are my first thoughts.

When I regain my composure, it dawns on me why he did this.

In retrospect, I remember indications of memory loss much, much earlier . . . like the time he came home from the office in the middle of the afternoon and just lackadaisically strolled around the house. It was totally unlike Hank, but I thought little of it at the time. I was just annoyed because he kept bothering me as I sewed.

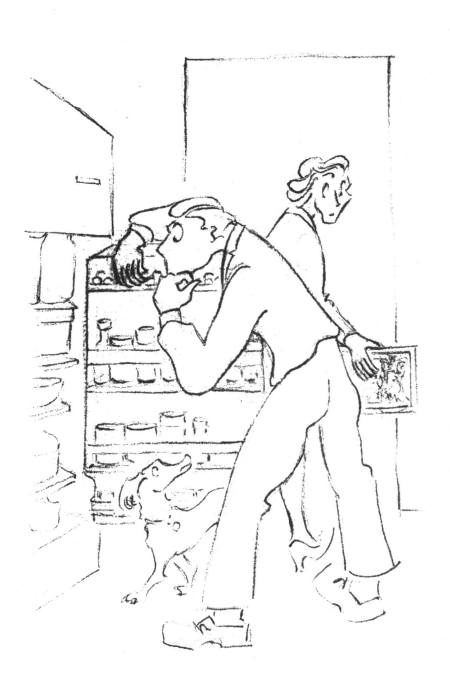

Third Year Spring, Sun City West

Our Sun City West house is ready. We take possession in late May. Hank is delighted at the prospect of calling this warm place "home" in winter.

Hank's determined we will have a citrus grove in our backyard. He pounds through the almost impenetrable layer of caliche to dig a hole so big that neighbors wonder if he'll disappear in it. He wants to make sure our little ten-gallon grapefruit is well started in life.

We're told it takes at least three years for citrus trees to bear fruit. This tree is so emaciated we doubt it ever will.

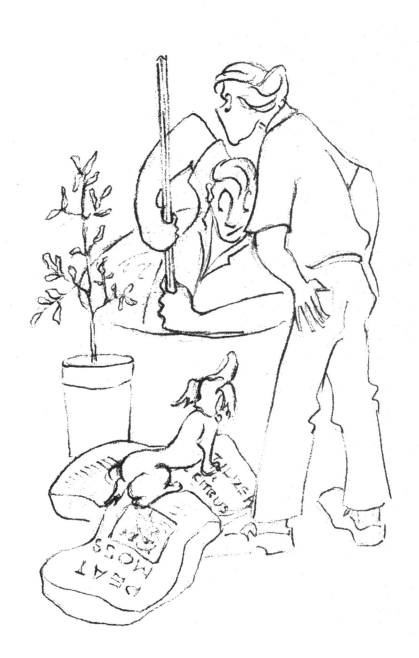

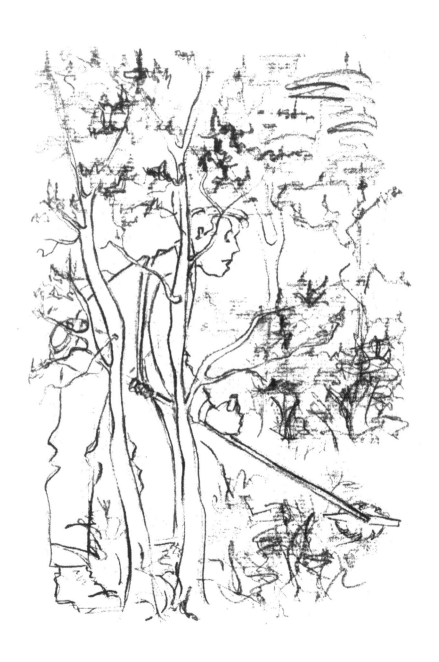

Third Year Summer, Cape Cod

When Hank goes out to clear the woods, he does it with a vengeance. It's hard labor. Hank stays with it for hours.

I worry about his using so lethal a weapon as his brush cutter, but his doctor says, "Would you rather have Hank leave this world doing something he loves doing, or have him take the long road out?"

Is there a choice?

Hank insists I take over the accounts . . .
pay the bills, etc. He's tired of the whole
business. I hate him for this, at first. Then I
actually begin to like it. In my innocence, I get
overconfident and consider that handling household
finances is very simple. When I come to my senses,
and realize I'm not quite as smart as I thought I was,
it's too late to ask Hank. He can no longer help.

I grit my teeth, do my best, but make some
very costly mistakes. How I wish I had paid more
attention to Hank's expert advice.

In my dilemma I welcome ideas from helpful
friends. One suggests selling languishing assets
while I can still take capital losses. I'll ask my
accountant.

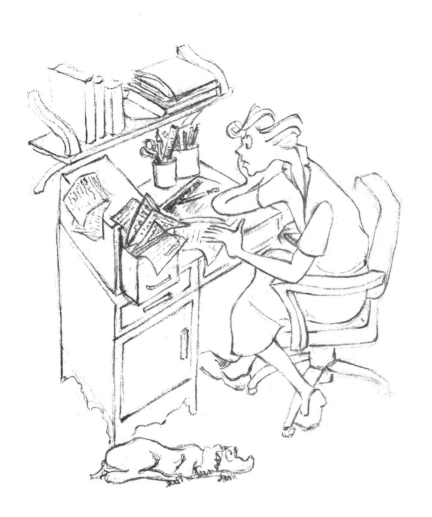

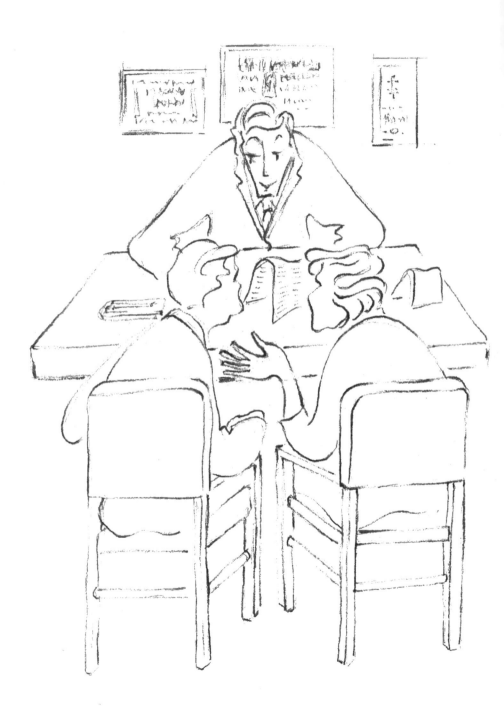

Third Year Fall, Sun City West

R ealizing we MUST get our affairs in order, we go through three lawyers, spend what seems, and is, a fortune, and finally locate one who seems to have OUR interests at heart.

After months of agonizing disenchantment, our wills, living wills, funded living trusts, and powers of attorney are signed. I breathe easier.

Both Hank and I are in good physical health, so unless something unforeseen happens, we should be adequately covered.

In all probability, getting our paperwork in order is one action we have taken early enough.

Fourth Year Winter, Sun City West

The ham radio tower belonging to one of Hank's more corpulent operator friends needs adjusting. While Hank waits for his own tower to arrive, he's on call.

Hank is agile as a monkey as he climbs to the top of the fifty-foot tower. Hanging there, he skillfully fine tunes the antenna.

Sometime later, when Hank's own tower arrives, the whole male population gathers to witness the installation. Veron, our neighbor, is the prime mover. For months he has been putting the whole thing together, with Hank sort of looking on.

I smile as I watch my Hank, full of importance, acting as if he's directing the whole operation.

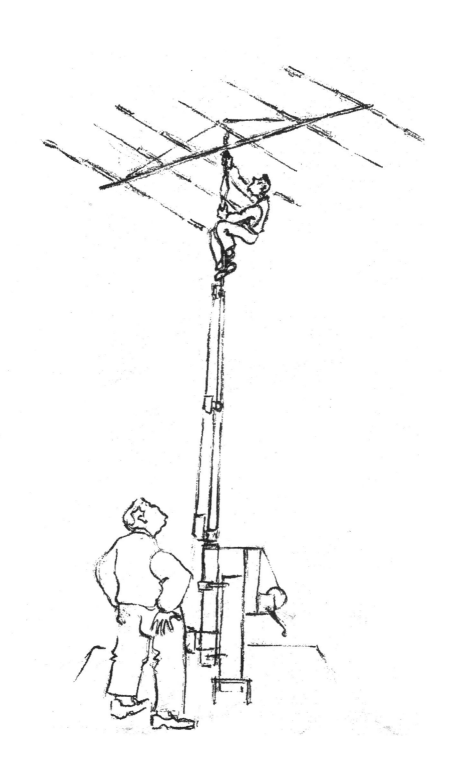

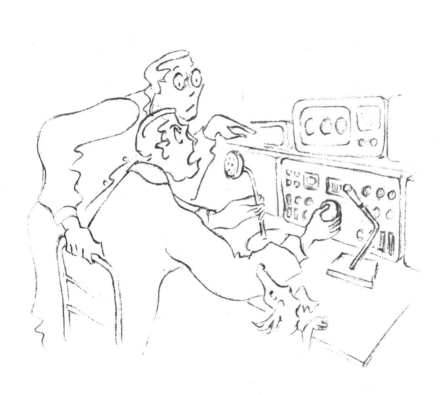

Fourth Year Spring, Sun City West

Hank gets on the air, "W 1 Sail Zed Sail. CQ. CQ. CQ. Calling CQ. Come in someone!" Hank tries valiantly to operate in the efficient manner to which he's been accustomed for almost fifty years . . . since he got his license at age fourteen! Now he keeps breaking into ongoing conversations, getting his and incoming call letters garbled, operating outside his transmission band. He just can't seem to get it right, despite compassionate help from proficient ham, friend and neighbor Al Fischer.

Angry voices and perplexed queries keep coming through. I'm embarrassed to think of hams at the other end wondering, "What's this I'm hearing?" I try and try to help Hank man the transmitter, but only make things worse.

Frustrated, upset and angry at both himself and me, he tries transmitting less and less. Finally, he gives up altogether.

I feel awful about this. Ham radio has been one of Hank's greatest joys for as long as I've known him.

As part of our house beautification project, Hank moves over three thousand pounds of flagstone, plus sand, cement and patio block, from the street where all the stuff is dumped to the back where I'm in charge of patio "layout."

We work daily in the cool of the morning: 5 to 10 a.m., then collapse. It takes us six weeks to complete, but neither of us has ever been in better physical shape. We can run up Squaw Peak like antelopes. Not bad for age sixty-four!

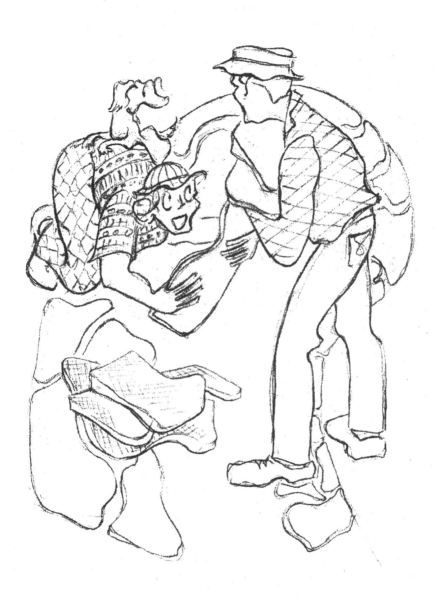

Fourth Year Summer, Cape Cod

Though Hank loved his civil engineering days as an overseas operations manager for an oil company, he always looked forward to retirement. He dreamed of having the time to read, do woodworking, keep bees, do some planting, get on the air with his ham radio rig. Now, unable to do much of anything, he begins to feel inadequate, suffers periods of depression, wants to get back to work, do anything, go anywhere . . . even to Saudi Arabia, which, despite his tolerance for heat, he always thought was TOO hot.

He's always been my mainstay . . . so sure of himself and his direction. When he falls apart, I flounder.

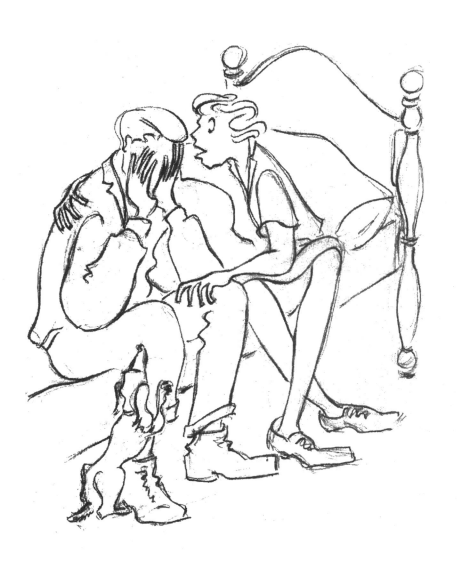

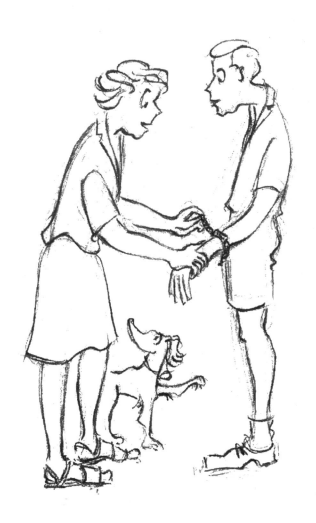

Hank has been gone for several hours. I can't find him anywhere. I begin to panic. Where can he be? I don't even know where to start looking for him.

The police find him striding gaily along the main road pushing a grocery cart. When they deposit Hank at the door, he's so unconcerned you'd think he'd never left home.

This makes me realize Hank needs permanent identification attached to him. I have a massive silver bracelet inscribed with all the pertinent details. I just hope he won't object to wearing it. Amazingly enough, he never seems to notice.

We have a leftover ticket from one of our travels . . . just enough to get one person to Alaska and back. It seems the ideal time for Hank to visit our son, Tucker, who works on the pipeline there.

Can Hank make this trip alone? In my enthusiasm to have "my men" holiday alone together, I decide to let Hank run this risk, half-pretending his problem doesn't exist.

When I'm told Hank will have a stopover in Seattle, I begin to have second thoughts. But I take a deep breath, cross my fingers, check his ID bracelet, tie identification tags to everything and HOPE.

I spend some very anxious moments until Tuck calls from Anchorage to say Hank made it. Getting "my traveler" back home won't be a problem. In two weeks, Tucker will come back to the Cape with him.

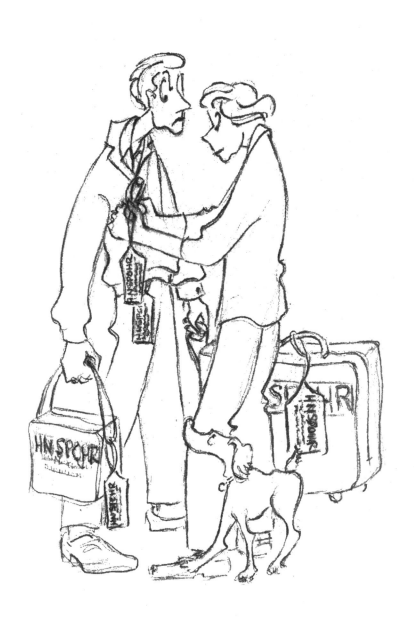

Hank has always had a fetish about water safety. He's about to take the Jeffersons, our weekend visitors, on a sightseeing tour around the little island on which we live. Suddenly he decrees, "Put the oars and life preservers on shore!"

Everyone is aghast. Neither our small boat nor its motor is wholly dependable. Nothing will sway Hank from his adamant decision.

Why is he so irrational? He's acting like a spoiled six-year-old. *What's gotten into him?* I think to myself.

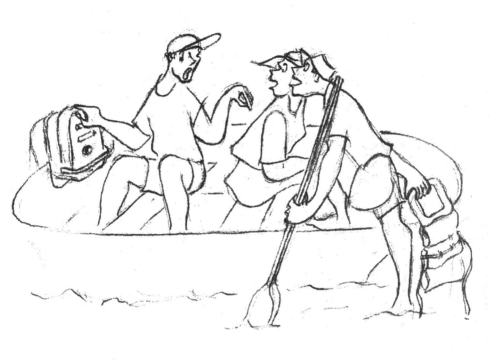

Fifth Year Spring, New Zealand

I think we'd better do the things we'd like to do while Hank still can. We fly off to New Zealand with one hundred and two other RVers. Our flock of little motor homes splits up into small groups to swarm over these two magnificent islands.

Until we get our "land legs," driving on the left is somewhat hazardous for us and anything in our way.

Hank has no qualms. He maneuvers every precipitous climb, hairpin turn, slippery metal (unpaved) road, and narrow one-way railroad/car bridge with as much dexterity as he did years ago when we lived in countries where people drive on the left side of the road.

Urban areas involve traffic, street locations and frequent turns. Hank leaves that up to me. I've never driven this size RV. In fear and trepidation, I try my hand at the wheel. It's fun!

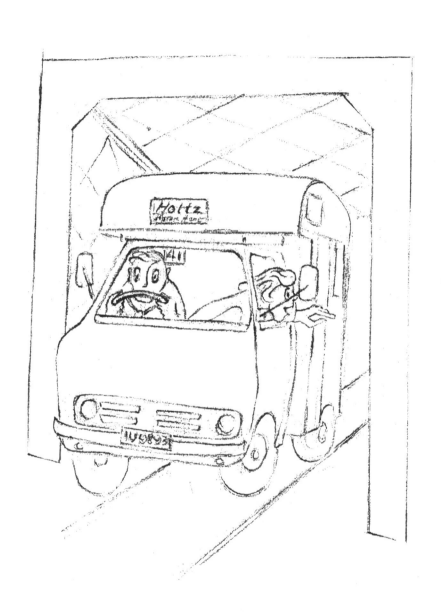

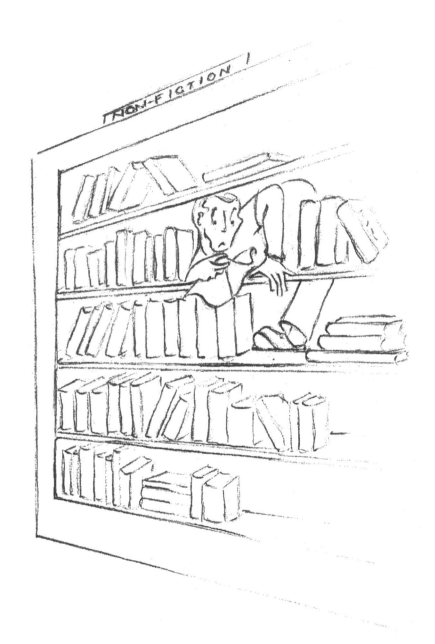

Fifth Year Spring, Sun City West

Each Saturday Hank putt-putts to the library on his little Lambretta. He volunteers there as "dust man."

"I'm small. I can get into places no one else can," he boasts.

He never did have any delusions of grandeur.

In addition to the library job, I look for an outdoor activity to help fill Hank's days. Remembering his love for all growing things, I volunteer our services as gardening crew at our property owners' headquarters. We operate rather successfully for several seasons, then Hank loses interest and I haven't the brawn to do heavy cutting and pruning.

My friend Elaine comes along when we go to practice our bowling skills. Hank gets so angry at his inability to "do it right." Elaine, who doesn't know about Hank's AD, asks me afterward if Hank needs psychiatric help.

As Hank has always been upset when he didn't live up to his own expectations, this bowling behavior doesn't strike me as excessive. But I'm embarrassed and unnerved to realize suddenly how Hank must appear to strangers and even to friends like Elaine.

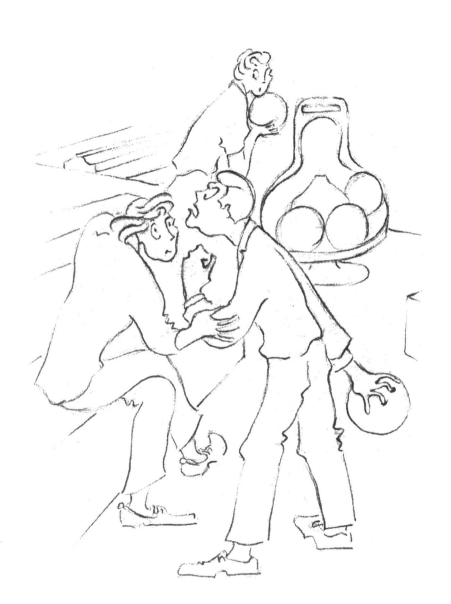

Fifth Year Spring, En Route

As we travel back and forth between Arizona and Massachusetts we're really done in each evening when we finally find a campground. Still, Noni and I have to be on the alert to be sure Hank goes to the proper washroom door, and gets back to the proper camper . . . ours, not a stranger's.

I'm very uneasy whenever he is out of sight and find myself secretly checking on him as I would a wandering four-year-old.

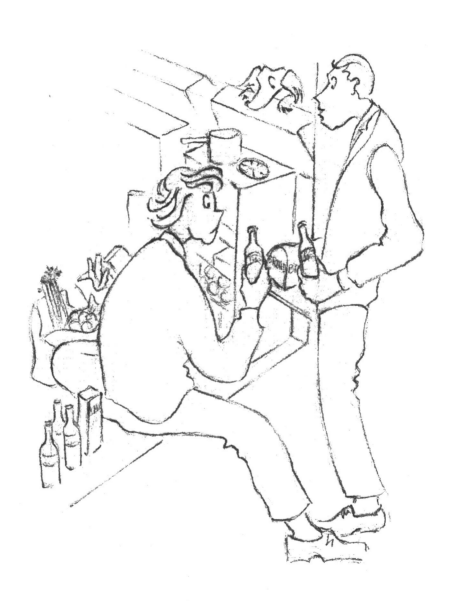

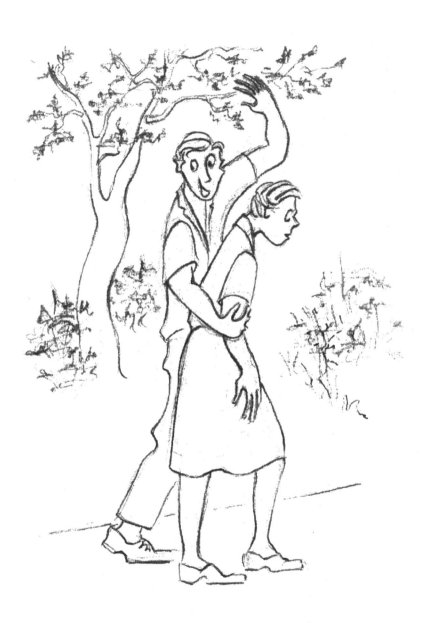

Fifth Year Summer, Cape Cod

Florence and Ed Powers have been regular summer visitors for a number of years. Florence can no longer understand or do much of anything. Alzheimer's has taken its toll.

Since the beginning, Ed has cared for Florence at home with minimum help. He's always tried to make her feel important. He's been unbelievably patient, and always loving.

Seeing these two together has been a good example for me. With Hank several steps behind Florence, it's been helpful, too. I'm somewhat better prepared for each new change, but it's frightening to know that this is what is in store for us.

Surprisingly enough, Hank has never seemed to relate his problems to Florence's. I doubt if he could now.

As we wave them off, I realize this is probably Florence's last good-bye. Tears are very near the surface. For them, for us.

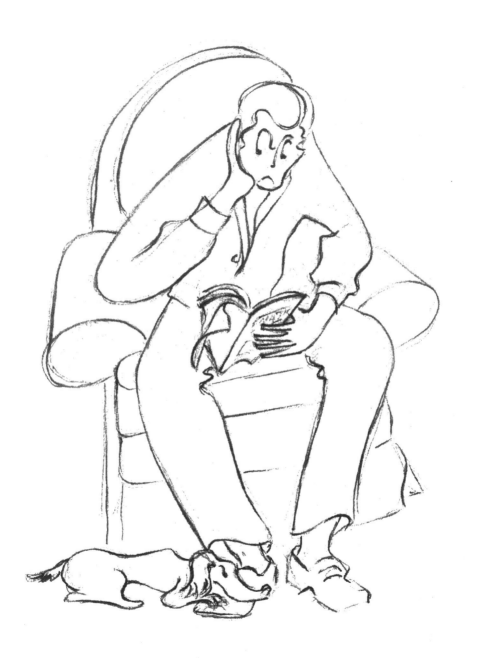

It's hard to realize how absolutely essential memory is to functioning as a rational human being. Watching Hank lose one ability after another is devastating.

He's always been an avid magazine reader . . . never without one in his hand or pocket. Now he goes through all the motions but never gets beyond page one.

He can be in the middle of his own living room and decide, "Let's go. Let's go home. Let's go. I want to go home." It's useless to argue with him because it only angers him. He's only reasonable in short spurts now.

Fifth Year Fall, Sun City West

Frequently we go to The Rec Center for Saturday night dances. Hank's fine on the dance floor but conversationally somewhat chaotic. Friends look askance when he loudly interrupts with a totally irrelevant comment. I find myself trying to cover up, protect him. I can't seem to tell them why. If Hank doesn't know, should they? I'm not yet ready to "go public."

How I wish these people had known Hank when he was really Hank.

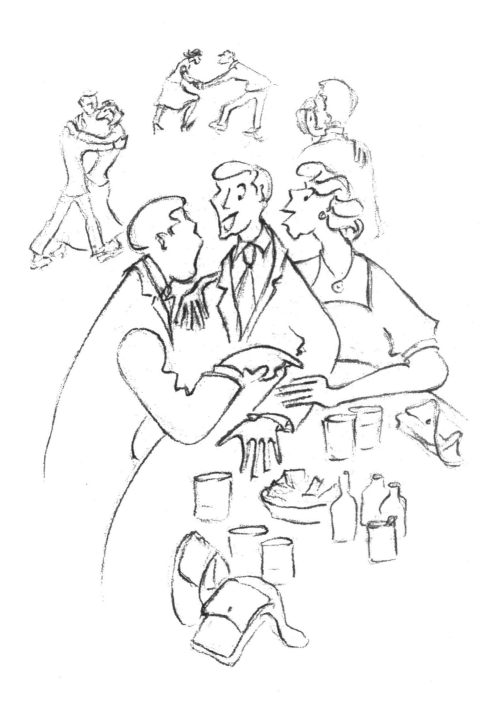

Points to Remember

1. If a major move is necessary, consider the patient's needs.

2. Remember to allow for mistakes due to illness.

3. Learn about family finances before it is too late.

4. Get your legal affairs and wills in order.

5. Make sure all necessary papers are signed.

6. Physical labor is good for the mind as well as the body.

7. Be prepared for attacks of frustration.

8. Provide identification bracelet or tags.

9. Don't put off visiting loved ones.

10. Plan a vacation according to current ability, patient's and yours.

11. Find suitable volunteer work for patient and caregiver to do together.

II

We Go Public

THE SIXTH YEAR

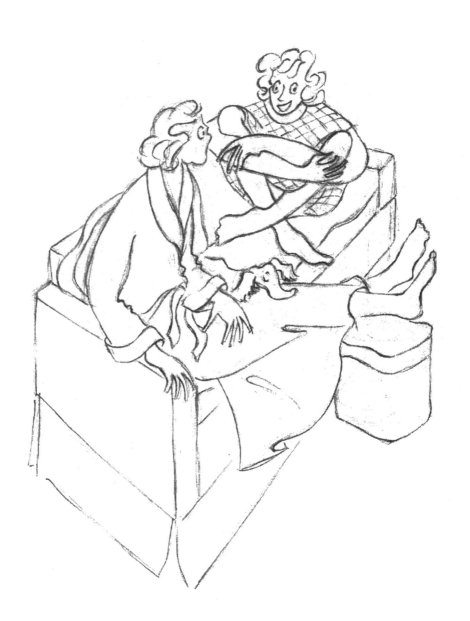

Sixth Year Winter, Sun City West

Friends can't help but notice that something is wrong with Hank. One will guardedly ask, "Has Hank been ill?" Another, "Has Hank had a stroke?" If I name the problem, I'm afraid I'll get the patronizing or "Oh! So sad!" reactions.

Kate, our daughter, here for Christmas, sets me straight. "You owe it to your friends and to Dad," she says, "to admit the truth."

Reactions, once the news is out, are interesting. Our neighbor Veron says, "Hank could not have lost all his expertise unless something was drastically wrong. Alzheimer's explains his present condition."

Others, good friends included, seem to have a father, mother or ancient aunt to whom they compare Hank. Some divulge useful, helpful information.

Mostly, though, it's hard to take. This is not someone from another era we're talking about. This is a contemporary. This is my HUSBAND! I feel we are being put into some antique category. This really hurts.

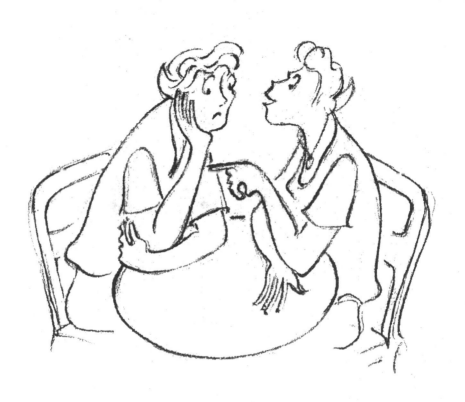

I go to an Alzheimer's support group meeting. Sharing experiences, problems, solutions does help.

I meet a very special elderly couple there who are an inspiration to all of us. For many years, the husband has, without help, been caring for his wife.

Putting his arm around his wife, the man says, "She always wants to go home to her mother's. Her mother's been gone for fifteen years. But I say, 'O.K. Let's go.' And we do . . . go anywhere."

Then he says, "We travel the world, too. Each morning I say, 'Honey, where will we go today? India? Japan? Portugal?' And off we go . . . by car, by foot, any way, just go. It makes her happy."

He adds, "I never argue with her. She doesn't like it."

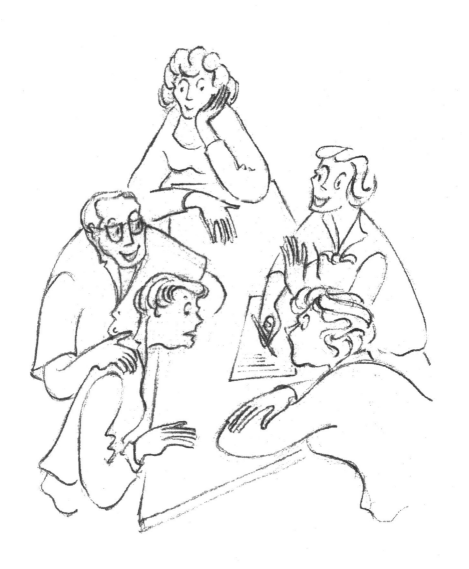

Sixth Year Spring, Sun City West

Our son Tucker, visiting us from Alaska, has been reading John Le Carré nonstop and is caught up in the spy ethic. He's convinced his father was a "spook" during the six years he worked in Vietnam.

Come to think of it, Hank did make several mysterious "business" trips to the States and, as a civilian, frequently traveled in upcountry Vietnam. Most of his military friends were in intelligence. Tucker might be right.

Tucker tries to nudge specific information out of his Dad and catches enough glimpses to confirm his suspicions. But Hank is so incoherent, nothing can be proven.

We regret lost chances to reconstruct the blank patches of Hank's life, about which he spoke so little when he was still able to communicate.

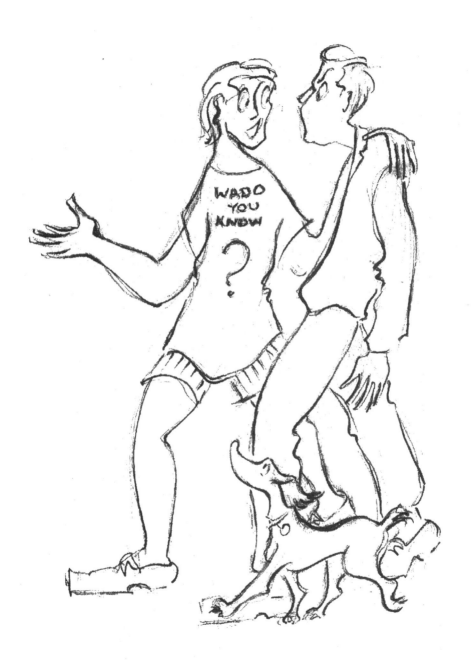

I begin to think we should go into a life-care facility. Hank is mobile, and we can be accepted now. Later, I discover the one we signed up for is financially shaky. The dining room depresses Hank. It depresses me too, if I want to be honest.

We book into another, put our house on the market and wait.

My big reservation is the "no pets" rule. Hank is so dependent on and fond of Noni that I'm not sure how to handle this.

Concerned friends strongly advise against this move, reinforcing my underlying doubts about the change. Just before our move-in date, we take our house off the market and look for alternative solutions.

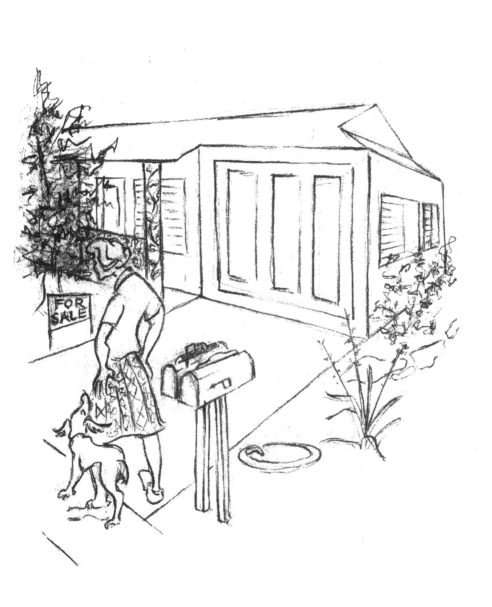

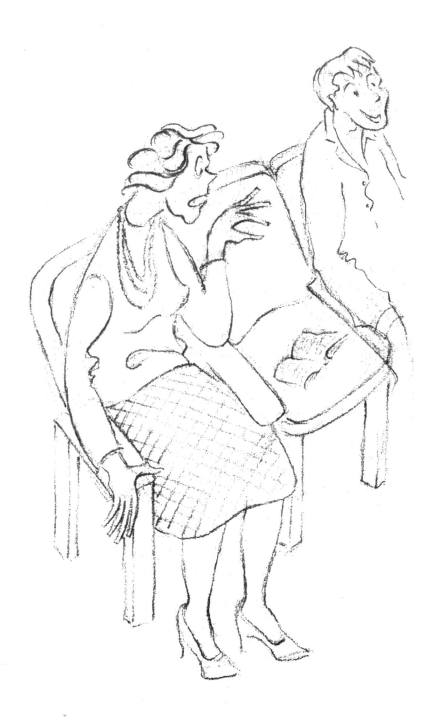

Sixth Year Spring, Cruising

Hank has seen our son in Alaska. It's about time I did, too. Deciding to do THIS trip in style, we book passage on the Cunard Princess.

One evening as we cruise north, we take in a movie. Halfway through the film, I realize Hank is gone! I panic! Where is he?

I race through lounges, decks, the bar, the dining room and night club. No Hank!

After a long, futile search, I pick my way down through an interminable maze of halls and stairways toward our steerage stateroom, agonizing all the way over what to do next.

When I arrive, there's Hank, asleep and snoring.

Our dining room steward, I find out later, piloted him home!

Sixth Year Summer, Cape Cod

Like an ornery three-year-old, Hank's greatest delight is to stand right in front of the TV when I'm REALLY engrossed in some program. He seems not to watch anything. Even an Alzheimer's program makes no impression. He just wants attention, I guess.

Dialing and answering the phone gets to be an impossible puzzle, but wanting him to do whatever he can as long as he can, I try to maintain a "hands off" policy. When he is trying so hard, it takes a lot of self-control not to do the job for him.

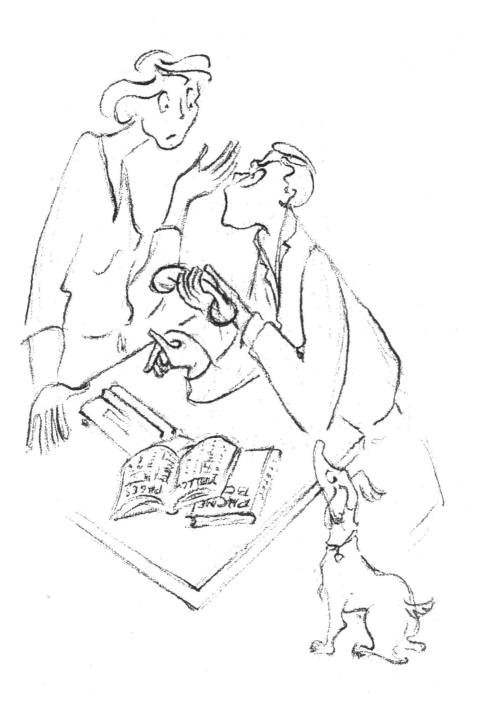

Sixth Year Fall, En Route

We stop to sign the visitors' book at one of the museums we visit as we mosey across the country.

I wonder what's taking Hank so long and find him agonizing over his signature, an illegible scrawl!

As I look at the register it suddenly dawns on me . . . thank heavens we established powers of attorney some time ago and signed all our legal documents.

I want to cry when I realize how many of Hank's abilities are gone.

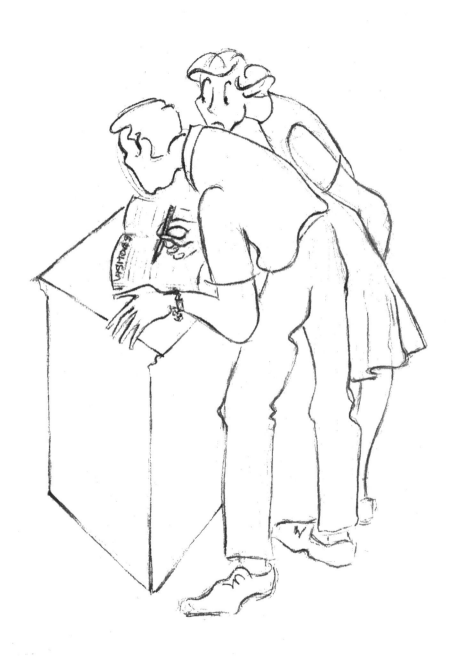

This is sure to be the last time we motor across the country. I'm doing ninety percent of the driving . . . more than I can or want to do.

Near Amarillo, we descend into a canyon to find another of Texas' magnificent state parks. Going down, I revel in the scenery and look forward to a refreshing night's sleep. Down in the canyon, I look up! How will we get out? I can't negotiate steep grades. Can Hank? I spend a frighteningly sleepless night wondering what to do. Call AAA to haul us out?

Morning comes at 5 a.m. I'm exhausted. Hank is as fresh as the proverbial daisy.

"What do you think about driving up out of here?" I tentatively suggest.

"Let's go!" says Hank.

Hands on the wheel, he's confident. He takes every twist, turn and gear shift like a pro. Zoom! Up and out and on we go. I can't believe it! How can he be so efficient one minute and devoid of reason the next?

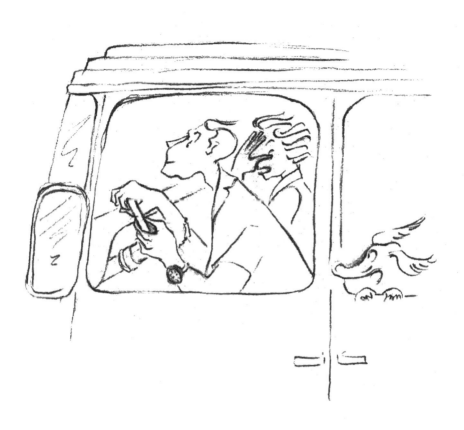

Sixth Year Fall, Sun City West

Hank is our mail collector. When he gets greedy and collects our neighbor's as well as ours, something has to be done. As I might have known, our neighbors are most cooperative and understanding.

The Postal Service, however, is bogged down in red tape. Only after prolonged negotiations and several weeks of paperwork are we allowed to move our neighbor's mailbox to the other side of his house. It works like a charm.

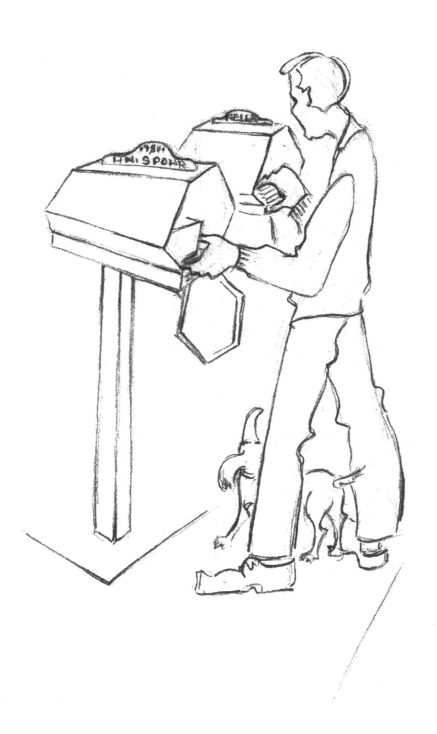

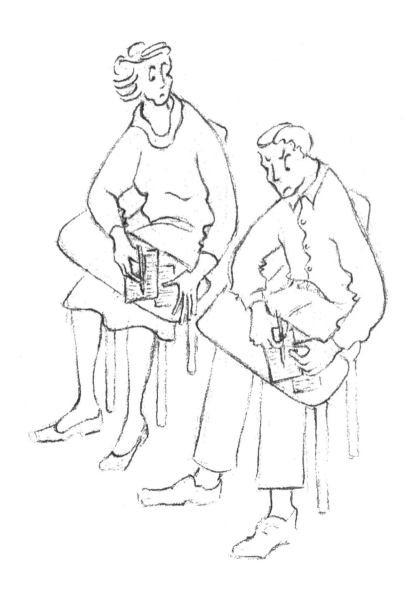

Selling our "Yellow Bird" camper is a trauma for us. When we go to transfer the title, we find that both our driver's licenses are four months in arrears. We have to renew them pronto. Because each of us had a minor traffic violation during the past year, Arizona law requires us to retake the written test.

I get through the test reasonably well, but Hank's having trouble. What's the matter with me? Now I'M being irrational. I should have known he couldn't do it.

Hank's driving days are obviously over. This is going to be very difficult.

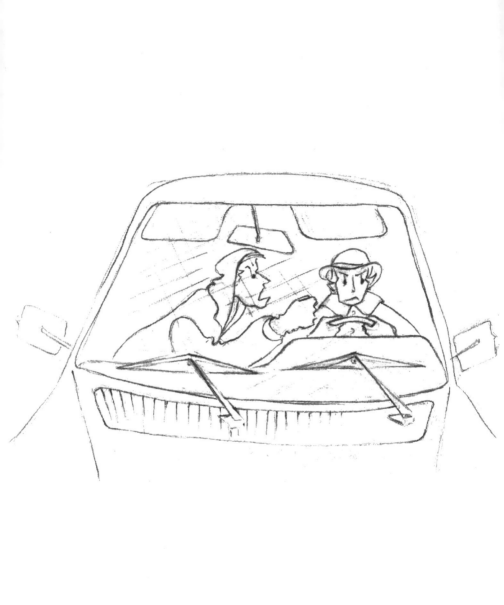

Sixth Year Christmas, Sun City West

The transition from driver to passenger is painful. Mostly Hank accepts my reasoning because I am normally the navigator. "Isn't it easier for me to drive? And isn't it nice just to sit back and relax?" When he rebels and insists on driving, things get a bit dicey.

Going to Grand Canyon for Christmas, we follow friends. Hank decides it is time he takes the wheel. I try to convince him that we will lose our friends if we stop to change drivers. Hank isn't buying any of "that garbage."

He shouts and shakes his fist at me, "You don't know what this does to a man. You're selfish and you don't care how I feel," and on and on. I cringe under the tirade but cling grimly to the wheel and DRIVE.

Coming home, women travel in our car. Men, with Hank in the back seat, travel in the other. This solves the problem for the moment at least.

Points to Remember

1. *Be open about Alzheimer's disease. Hiding it does not help.*

2. *Join an Alzheimer's support group for understanding and care.*

3. *Gather family information early. Memory loss obliterates the past.*

4. *If a life-care facility, a senior residence, nursing home or any other facility is being considered, carefully check its viability and financial stability.*

5. *Accept behavior similar to two- or three-year-olds as normal for AD patients.*

6. *Innovative solutions can eliminate many problems.*

7. *Be diplomatic yet firm with the AD patient when it becomes impossible for them to drive.*

8. *Remove the patient from situations that can cause frustrations.*

III

Finding Help

THE SEVENTH YEAR

Seventh Year Winter, Sun City West

Hank lands in the hospital with an unidentified ailment. A battery of tests turns up nothing.

I leave him to go hear Itzhak Perlman in concert at the Sundome. I come back rejuvenated only to find Hank immobilized. He's furious.

"What are you doing to me? Get me out of here!"

The hospital wants him gone, too.

As he is being discharged, his doctor tells me, "You'll have to make some other arrangements for your husband."

"What do you mean? A nursing home?"

"Yes," replies the doctor.

"Permanently?"

"Yes."

This is a shocker. I can't quite face that yet.

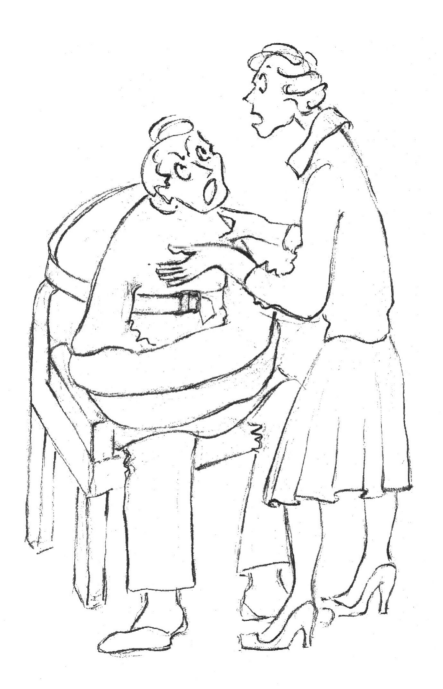

I wonder how Hank will react to a day care center? I get him there on the pretext that we can volunteer as helpers.

He does the morning's mild calisthenics and group activities in a fine, military manner. All goes so well, I leave just before lunch.

I go to pick him up and find the staff in a frenzy. Hank didn't go for any of the afternoon handicraft stuff. He walked off into the blue. Nothing would keep him happy after that.

Again he greets me with an angry, "What are you doing to me?"

Day care works so well for so many people, patients and caregivers alike. I wish it would work for us.

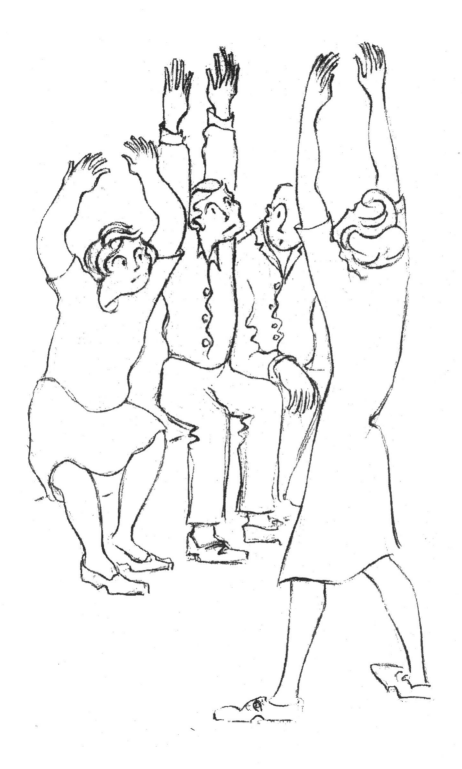

Seventh Year Spring, EPCOT Center

Exhausted after our first nonstop day at EPCOT, we fall into bed and into a sleep-to-end-all sleep.

At 3 a.m., I wake to find Hank's bed empty and the door ajar. Rushing to find him, I stop only to grab my coat. As I reach the hall, Hank is just disappearing toward the elevator. Almost simultaneously, our room door slams shut! No key! No shoes! Hair in disarray!

I finally recapture my charge, set him down by the door, and pray he'll stay put while I go in search of a pass key.

Heaven only knows what the night clerk thinks has happened. His knowing smile indicates he isn't going to believe the truth.

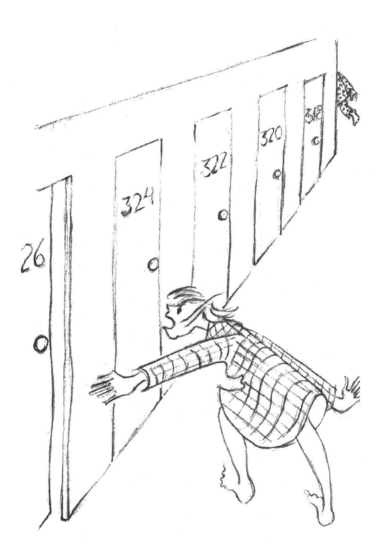

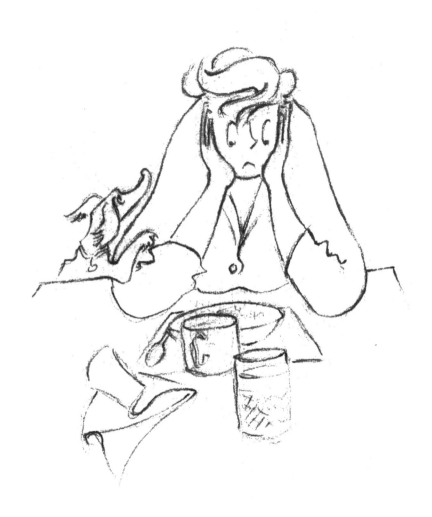

Seventh Year Spring, Sun City West

What to do next? Hank can no longer be left alone. I need help. A kind and wonderful friend, Dr. Tidwell, suggests that besides formal nursing home care, part-time, live-in and foster home care may be available.

Thank goodness our daughter, Deb, is here on a visit. We start exploring live-in help.

On the way to interview Paul O'Brien, our fourth candidate, Deb details all the things I must do. She suggests a contract that spells out obligations on both sides: time off, duties, salary.

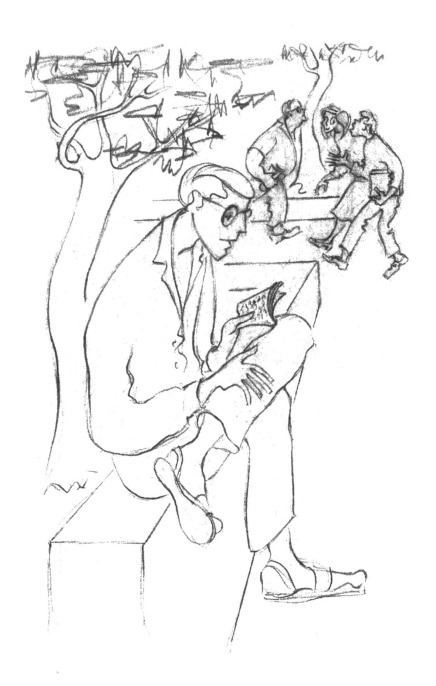

Paul impresses us. We like him. He's fifty, a graduate of Colorado School of Mines. Never married, not much family, few friends nearby. He's worked at a lot of different things in many different places: mining in Venezuela, lumbering in Canada, Salvation Army in Hawaii . . . you name it, Paul's done it. He is six-foot-two, well-built and personable.

Is Paul too good to be true? Desperate as I am, can I chance taking a complete stranger into the house? To our delight and amazement, Hank accepts Paul as if he's always been a member of the family.

D eb shocks me with, "Why don't you divorce Dad? Naturally, you'd still care for him, but it might eventually help financially."

She follows this with, "If Dad is hospitalized, really sick, would you allow support systems? Once authorized, you know, they can't be disconnected. Of course, you wouldn't withhold liquids, but what about food?"

These are disturbing questions. Our living wills should cover support systems. But divorce?

Deb, who loves her father deeply, is, nevertheless, concerned for me as well as her father. And because Alzheimer's may be hereditary, she's also concerned for herself and her three small sons.

Deb's been attending every workshop, lecture, and support group she can find. She's come up with some interesting tidbits: Alzheimer's victims maintain good health until their defenses are down and they contract something lethal, like pneumonia; the younger the victim, the shorter the illness; England has a very high incidence of Alzheimer's.

Deb's questions are valid. They make me THINK.

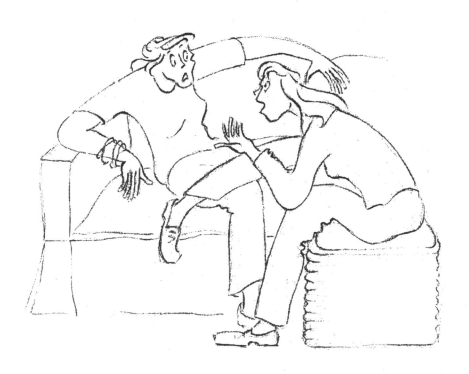

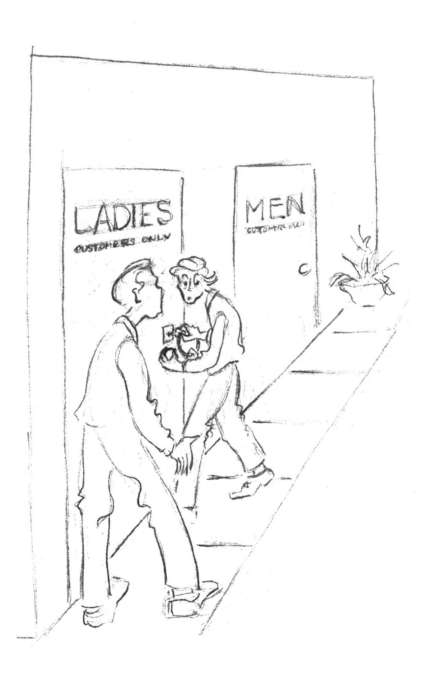

When we go out anywhere, we have to make frequent comfort stops because Hank is not completely dependable.

Since he can't manage rest rooms alone, I'm grateful for gas stations, especially when Paul is not with us. Usually we can use outside entrances for unisex pit stops.

I try to choose uncongested spots, disliking the quizzical expressions we receive after emerging "en deux" from the LADIES.

Seventh Year Summer, Cape Cod

It's barely a month since Paul arrived, and we're back on Cape Cod. We find the house just as Hank and I left it, in a mess. Furniture is piled in the middle of the living room. Books are all over the place. The room is ready to be painted. But the man who promised to do it has another job, so no time to work for us. There's no way we can settle down until that room is done.

Paul goes to work with a vengeance.

Hoping to keep Hank localized while he paints, Paul sets up a special "workshop" where he can check up on Hank every once in a while.

The unpainted shelves Paul puts out for Hank to finish painting never get done. Hank's quite content to stay in the "shop" but paints the ladder on which the shelves are set instead of the shelves. We end up with some very interesting green ladders.

Among other activities, Paul sets Hank to work "vacuuming" the shop. It hardly matters if he's plugged in or not.

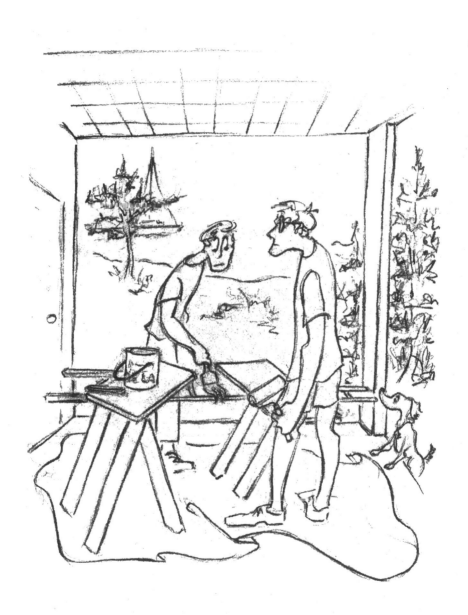

P aul fits Hank out with an empty wheelbarrow, a ploy to keep him busy and not "on a wander." Hank marches around the house so purposefully, Noni fears a collision. Scared though Noni is, Hank seems happily content with his new, "gainful employment."

When this fun pales and Paul isn't looking, Hank breaks out of his round-the-house wheelbarrow routine. He's halfway to the causeway when Paul discovers his charge is missing.

Off Paul goes at a brisk trot. Hank isn't hard to find with his brilliant barrow. Paul has painted all tools and shop equipment a vibrant, signal-corps orange!

"Well, I kind of like orange. It's a good color," says Paul.

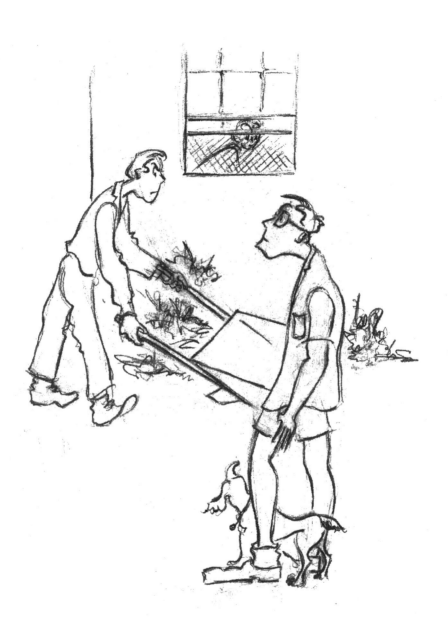

We have house guests. After dinner one night, Hank wanders off as usual. Suddenly he appears, clothes in hand, looking very pleased with himself. He's bare as the day he was born!

I'm anything but nonchalant as I nervously remove him from the living room. After the initial shock, the assembled guests regain a sort of uneasy composure.

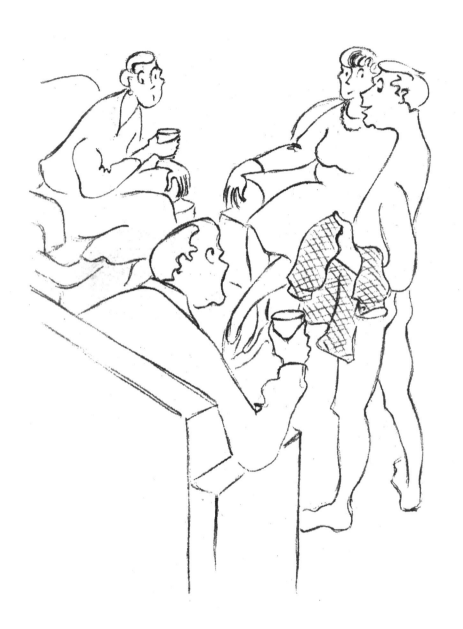

Our bedroom begins to smell like a latrine. I wake each morning to near-asphyxiation. Screens are raised. All the insect kingdom is holding court. Intensive research localizes the offensive odor in one corner. Try as we do, neither Noni nor I can ferret out the exact source.

Then shines the light: Hank, in failed efforts to find the bathroom, has been answering night calls of nature through the window. He's been carefully raising the screen, avoiding it as well as the carpet. But he hasn't been able to direct his fire accurately enough to miss the window frame.

A night light in the bathroom and hall, and a day's scrubbing, solve THAT problem.

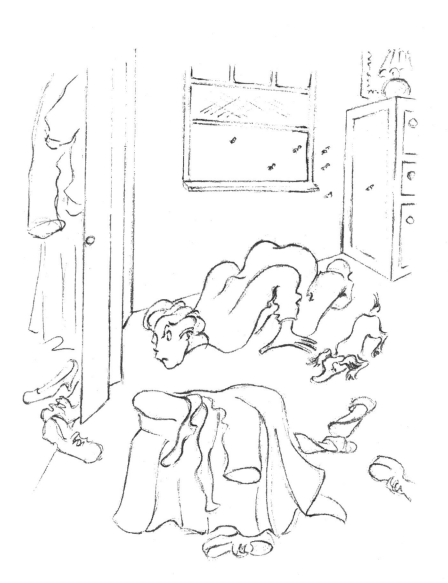

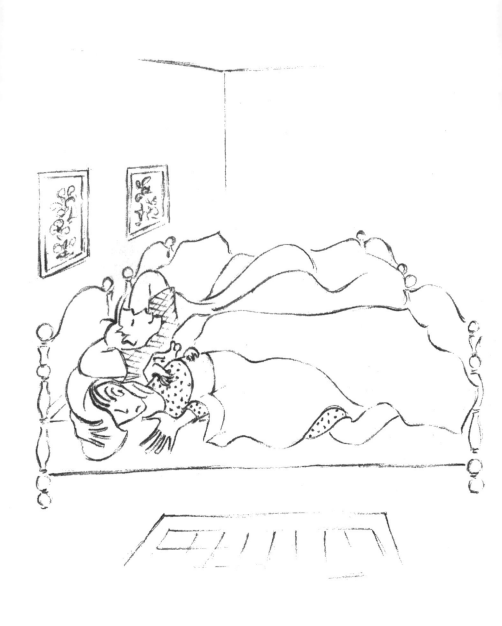

Things get pretty congested when Hank decides he likes my bed better than his. He happily preempts three-quarters of the available space. This causes a bit of a conflict. Noni considers my bed HER domain. I consider it MINE. Now Hank considers it HIS.

We push two single beds together to make one super-size king and THAT solves THAT.

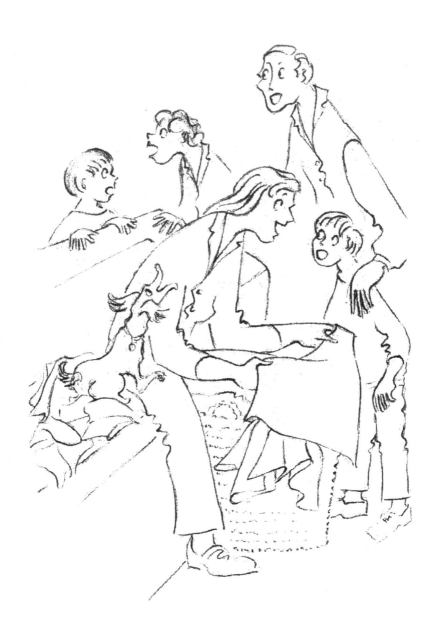

Deb's summer visits always add to life's confusion and joys. While she sorts laundry, she and her three boys burst into "Jesus Loves Me." Hank gets into the spirit of the thing with his own atonal, garbled version of the song. They all seem to like this "close" kind of harmony.

Deb reads to her Dad from his own well-worn Bible. She picks out the passages he, himself, underlined during the years when he read and studied so faithfully.

Hank's contented smile would indicate at least a glimmer of understanding. Maybe it's Deb's nearness and love that gets through to him.

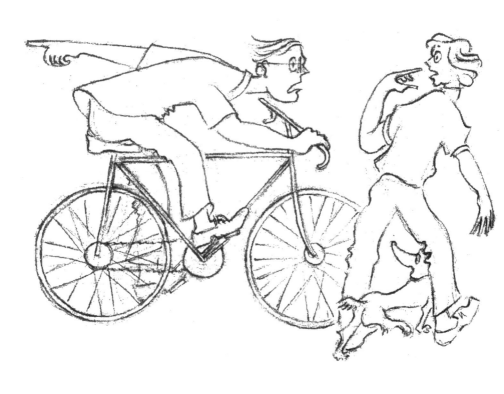

Seventh Year Fall, Sun City West

Back in Arizona, we have more problems. Hank keeps disappearing. Where has he gone? Before we call the posse, Paul goes one way, I go the other. Paul almost always finds the wanderer.

"I've done a lot of stalking in my time," he says.

To counteract this wandering, Paul devises such an impenetrable security system, it thoroughly baffles all of us. He invents an ingenious screen-door lock, using huge, plastic paper clips. Even Paul and I find it difficult to escape.

I'm thankful for one problem we do not have. Hank isn't a smoker. We've never had to worry about matches or forgotten lighted cigarettes as some other caregivers must.

Anyone who has problems with a smoker might try my friend Joan's imaginative solution. When her Mom, a smoker, asked for a cigarette, Joan said, "Mom, you stopped two years ago!" How easy that was!

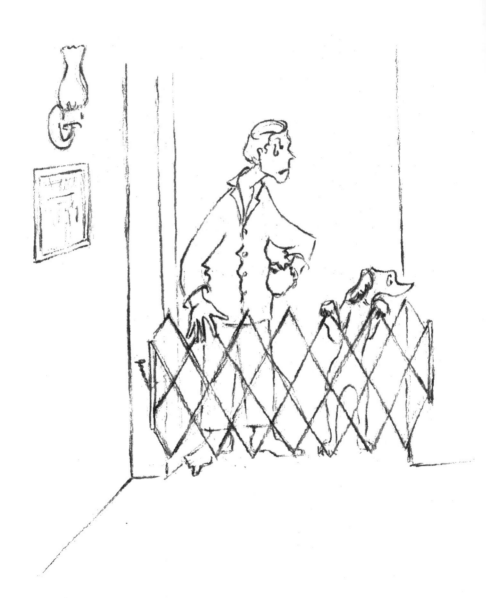

It's been years since Hank and I have been sexually close. I miss his touch, his physical nearness. Now Hank's restlessness leaves me sleepless and bone-weary. Any day when he's not too agitated or demanding I pen him someplace out of harm's way and take a nap.

At night a baby-gate does yeoman's service as both man- and dog-gate. It turns out to be just enough of a deterrent to keep both Hank and Noni from wandering into the Great Beyond.

The one thing Hank CAN and WILL do is walk . . . and walk Hank and Paul do, often ten miles a day. Paul goes armed with his recorder blaring political, religious, historical speeches. Hank marches ahead toting their carry-all with water bottle, extra clothes, etc.

The pack keeps Hank balanced and his hands occupied so that he doesn't fiddle with his clothes and tear off all his buttons.

Paul keeps a firm hand on Hank's shoulder. If he forgets and gets too engrossed in his tapes, Hank is likely to take a 180-degree turn toward nowhere.

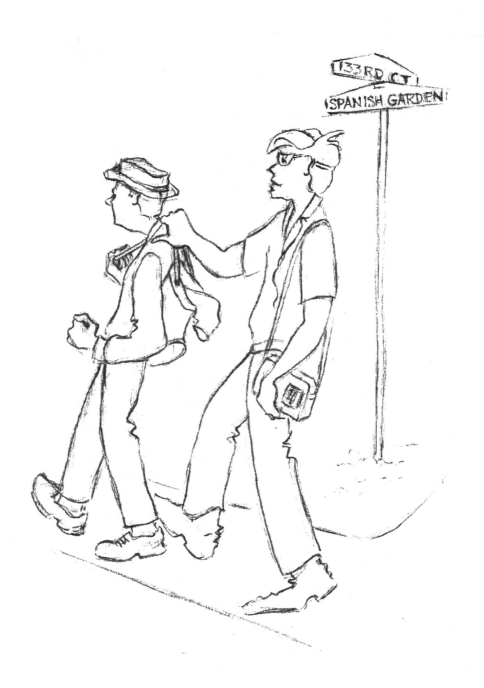

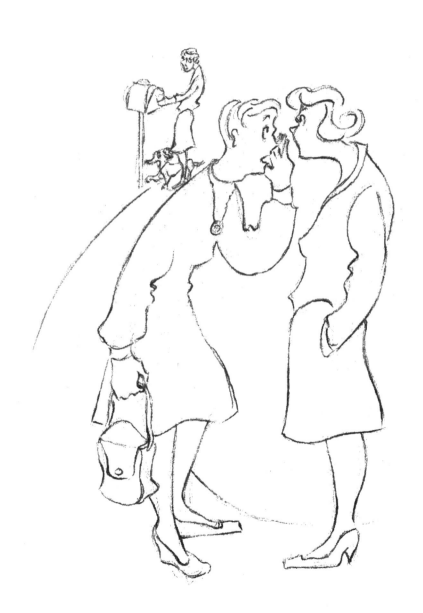

Some neighbors whisper, "How long will she keep him home?" There's no contest. At home, Hank is our only charge. We know what kind of attention he's getting, and medication, if any. For me, it's really easier. It requires no trekking back and forth to some institution to help with and check up on his care. Undoubtedly, it would even be less costly to keep Hank home than to choose any of the available alternatives.

I try not to waver when for some reason Hank pleads, "Help me! Please help me!"

I would if I could, but it's difficult to know what he wants since his speech is so garbled. I make all sorts of wild guesses, usually never hitting the mark.

It's heartrending to hear this cry for help from a man who used to say, "If you want something done right, do it yourself."

Points to Remember

1. For some, a day care center can work wonders.
2. Explore alternatives to nursing home care.
3. Live-in help can solve many problems.
4. Try to face issues early before a crisis occurs.
5. Be prepared for embarrassing AD behavior.
6. A sense of humor eases many awkward situations.
7. Invent repetitive tasks to keep patient busy and happy.
8. Add a security system and check locks on windows and doors.
9. Beware of smoking hazards.

IV

The Wanderer

THE EIGHTH YEAR

Eighth Year Winter, Sun City West

H ank keeps coming up from behind me without notice. He seems to want to stay close . . . too close for comfort.

He will grab me, or anyone who's handy, at the most unexpected moments.

"I love you, I love you. I do love you," he'll say, smiling broadly with tears welling from his eyes. Then angrily he'll say, "You are bad. Very bad. You bastard." This is kind of amusing, but makes me realize I couldn't live with constant verbal or physical abuse.

I'm not very sure Hank knows who I am.

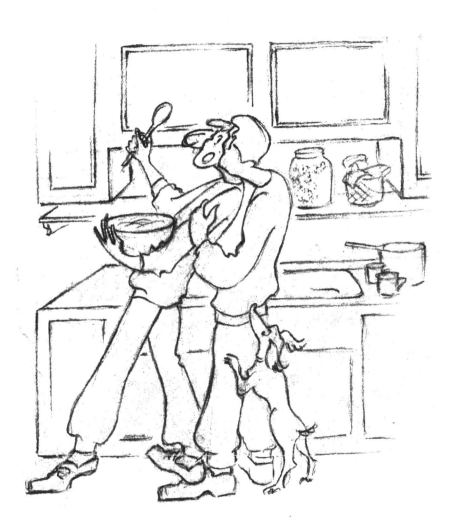

Hank develops a passion for cleanliness. He gets the grungiest rag he can find and scrubs everything in sight . . . even me.

This penchant for "cleaning" becomes rather embarrassing. Hank starts trying to "scrub" females, friends or strangers, in all-too-intimate places.

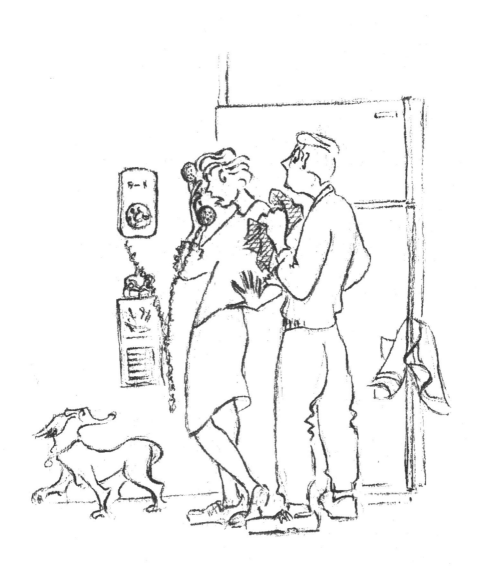

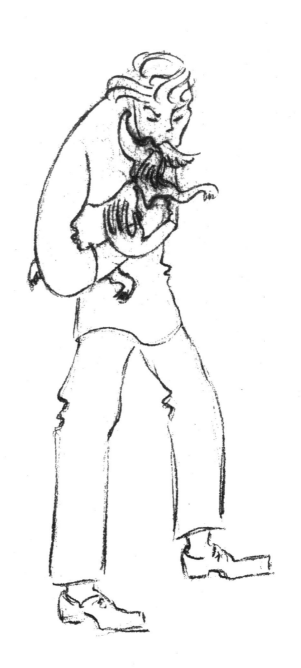

Hank's big activity is walking Noni. He takes her out so often she begins to wonder just what's expected of her. For a long time I have felt confident that Noni, even though she sees poorly and cannot hear, will bring them both home safely.

Neighbors begin to complain because Hank forgets to use our makeshift pooper-scooper. And, at fourteen, Noni's health is beginning to falter. When we go east again, I decide I can't put her through another tortuous plane ride confined in that little cage.

I take her for her last trip to the vet.

I feel awful.

I miss her.

Hank doesn't even know she's gone.

Eighth Year Summer, Cape Cod

Hank's wandering drives us crazy. It's almost impossible to keep track of him if he decides to go it alone. We're such characters around the supermarket that even management keeps an eye on him. The grocery boy almost always seems to have "just seen him."

When Hank escapes from the greenhouse while Paul and I are choosing our spring plants, or disappears into a flea market crowd, we have to enlist the services of our local police. They accept our S.O.S. calls with equanimity.

Occasionally, friends or even comparative strangers will call to say they've seen him going lickety-split into the woods. Then they'll often help us flush him out, even in the rain. I hate to impose, but I find there are a lot of compassionate people in this world.

It's time I take action. I'm told that there are some very successful 24-hour-a-day programs for finding victims who stray. The Alzheimer's Association's *Safe Return* is one, and often local police administer others. I must check them out.

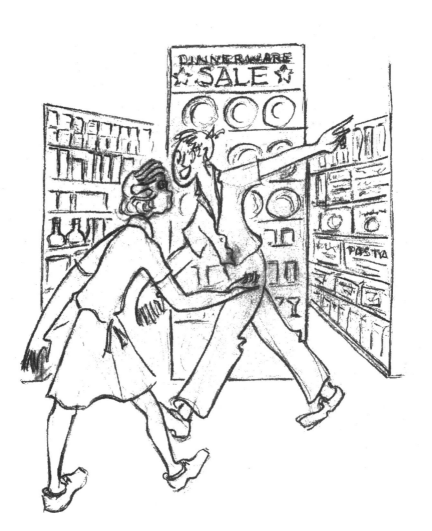

Deb and her children are visiting, and I'm concerned about keeping track of Hank while they are here. Our security system will be shot with a trio of boys, three, five and eight, going in and out of the house all the time.

I need not have worried. We notice that Hank has forgotten about our side entrance. We christen it "The Secret Door." "All Quiet" is the password. It's never to be used if Hank is looking.

This turns out to be the boys' favorite game. Cooperation is amazing!

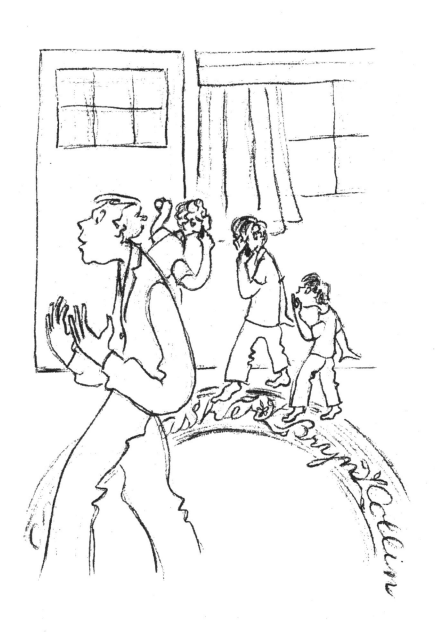

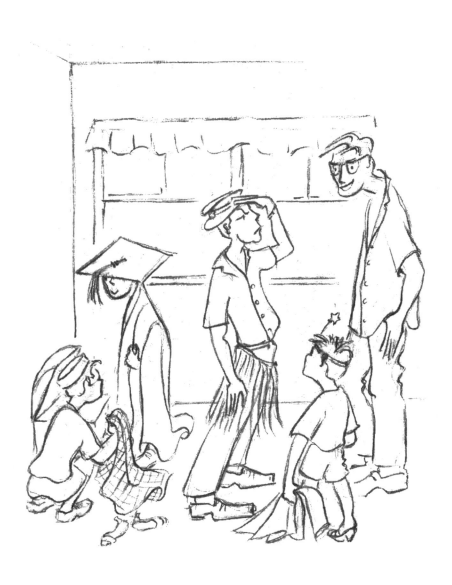

When rain keeps the troops indoors, Deb's kids discover the little costume trunk. Collin turns into a high-heeled angel, and Bryn into an Indonesian Tuan Besar (Important Man). When Asher unearths Hank's old Navy cap, Hank immediately appropriates it. He plops it on his head, comes smartly to attention, and gives a crisp, left-handed salute.

Says Paul, "Well, Hank must have been in the military."

Even when the grandkids aren't around, Hank puts on anything and everything he can find: his duck-billed cap, my skimpy shirt, Paul's XL pants and size 13 shoes. Dress up is a game with never ending possibilities.

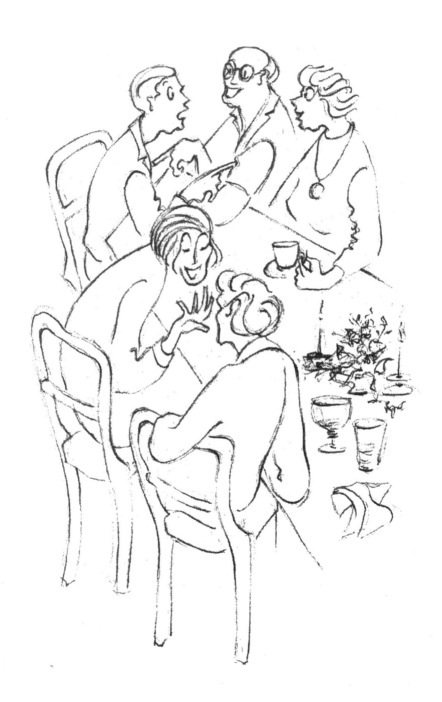

We have dinner with friends. One of the guests is a nonstop talker. He meets his match in Hank. Both talk, neither listens.

With Hank expounding his nonsense, and the guest going on about his experiences, they develop quite a rapport.

At first I'm afraid this will make the other guests uncomfortable. I need not have worried. They are all enjoying themselves so thoroughly they aren't even aware of this crazy interchange.

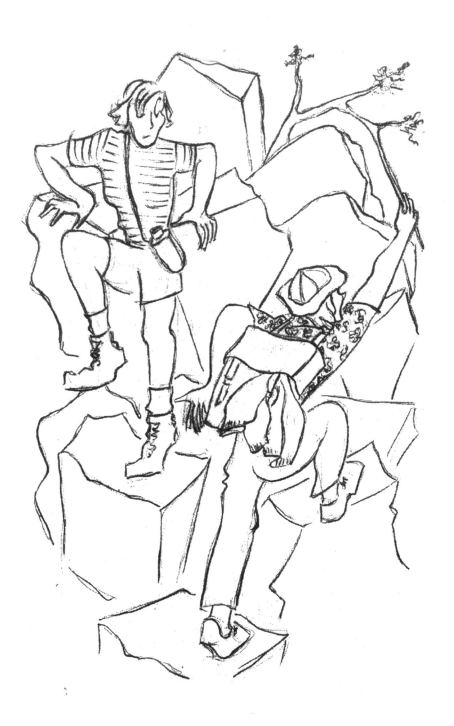

My Sister Mary takes over the distaff duties for Hank and Paul while I spend five days hiking a bit of Vermont's Appalachian Mountain Trail.

I can't help feeling guilty about taking off this way. I try not to think about him continually, but Hank is always in the back of my mind.

I'm not sure I can keep up with anyone, much less my athletic friend, Kit, ten years my junior.

Most of the time I wonder why I'm putting myself through this torture. Despite aches in every part of me, it's wonderful to get away and I begin to feel like I'm Kit's age, too. I'm actually enjoying myself.

Daughter Kate tells me the next time I undertake such a venture I'd better do myself the favor of getting in shape first. I couldn't agree more.

The day comes when I have to accept the inevitable. Hank needs to be diapered. Finding proper protection is a real poser. Regular or extra absorbency? Small, medium or large hip-size? How many? 10's? 30's? Just briefs with liners? An outside catheter? Bed pads: large or small? It's enough to make ME reach for a tranquilizer.

What's more, we use so many, the darn things could break the bank. Can I buy them in bulk?

And I thought I was through with diaper rash years ago!

At first, I'm really embarrassed about my waterproofing purchases and try to hide them. Camouflage proves all but impossible. Containers are huge and ungainly. No grocery bag will hold them. Few manufacturers provide handles to facilitate cartage. As time goes by, I realize I'm going to have to develop a nonchalant, so-what attitude about the whole thing but

It would be great
if God would create
creatures who need not eliminate.

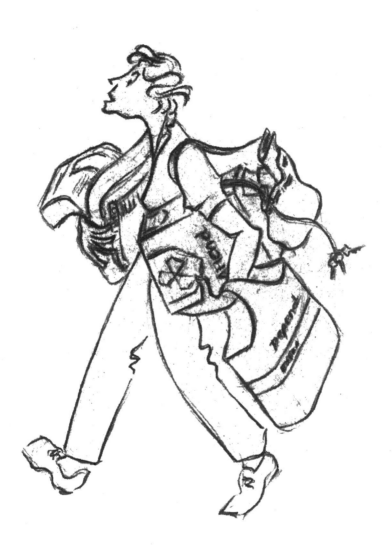

Eighth Year Fall, En Route

Fall . . . another flight back to Arizona. We're booked, two seats together and one single. I fear this may spell disaster, especially at mealtime. But a kind fellow traveler offers to shift. Three seats across with Hank in the middle are better for us AND for the other passengers.

Coping with nature's necessities on an airplane is, at best, difficult. I cannot imagine how tall Paul maneuvers in the minuscule, cubbyhole lavatories to help Hank. I envision some kind of accordion maneuver.

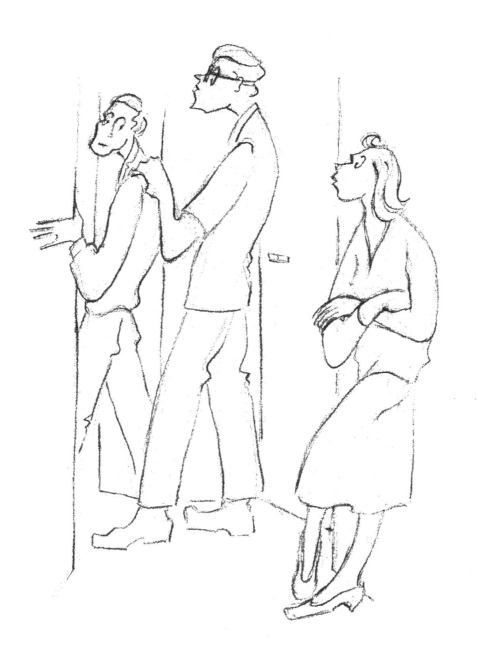

Eighth Year Fall, Sun City West

Hank is really pleased with himself when, after fidgeting with his shirt or sweater buttons, he manages to pull them off. Sewing them back on is my routine TV-watching activity.

I search for buttonless easy-on, easy-off clothing and find the jogging suit. This seems particularly appropriate for Hank, in light of his jogging history. I soon discover that, though the basic design is great, slip-ons are harder to use than zip-ups.

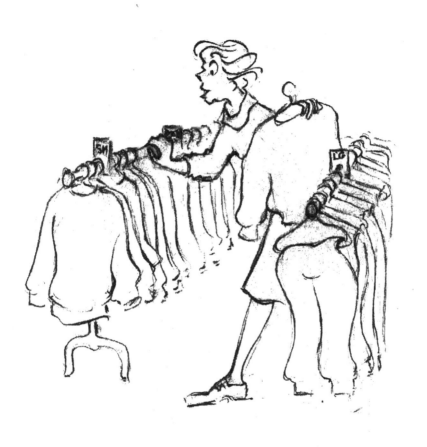

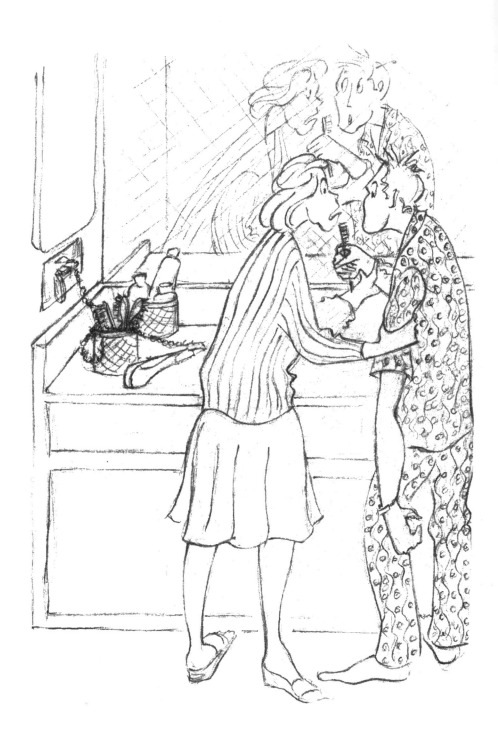

W e wonder what goes on in that head of Hank's. Around the end of October he starts agonizing, "I'm scared! I'm scared!"

Are there really witches on broomsticks flying around in his brain?

"That's OK," says Paul to soothe him. "What's Halloween for, anyhow?"

Hank's moods vary abruptly. Sometimes he acts downright ornery. He absolutely refuses to let me help him change into his pajamas. I get impatient and upset with him, even though I know he can't help it. Arguing just makes him more determined. Having sometimes to wait out his mood for several hours is exasperating.

I never expected to turn into a tonsorial artist. When Paul takes Hank to the barber, Hank is so fidgety that he's likely to end up with a rather weird haircut. The results aren't any better when I have to take over.

Another problem is dental hygiene. I barely manage to get Hank to brush his teeth by guiding his hand to his mouth. Even so, he never does a very complete job.

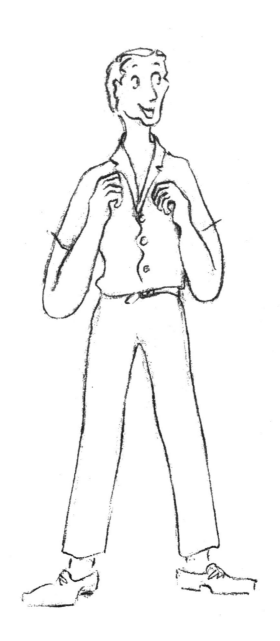

Though Hank doesn't react to much, sweets
are an exception. Ice cream is his first love,
cake his second. Both are rare treats in our
house. Any birthday, but especially his, is cause for
celebration, less for the occasion than for the perks.

He has most of his hair
his teeth are all there
his eyes and his ears are still good.
He eats mountains of food
he talks a blue streak
he walks miles every week.
At weight one-twenty-eight
he's in shape, really great.
He's just turned sixty-nine
he's still doing just fine.
There's not a thing wrong
    except
his memory is gone.

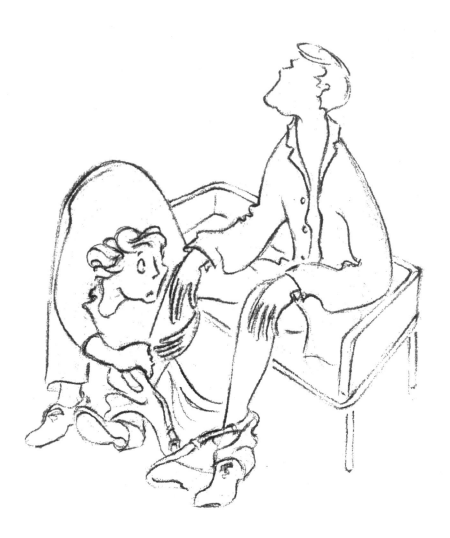

If an old friend asks, "What's my name, Hank?" Hank is baffled. Then the light slowly dawns. Hank, in his confusion, answers, "I'm Hank, Hank Spohr." He never seems to forget who HE is.

However, Hank's mixed-up brain seems to get everything in reverse: HE is SHE, UP is DOWN, and LEFT is RIGHT. In order to get his shoes off and pajamas on I have to touch the foot I want lifted.

Ninety percent of the time he lifts his right foot when I want him to lift his left. It takes a bit of persuasion to get it right. I have to be on the alert so as not to get showered, as I often was when dressing my two-year-old son.

Eighth Year Christmas, Sun City West

Hank is a study in perpetual motion. He barely stops to eat. En route, his constant chatter about nothing is better than a bell for determining his whereabouts. What is he thinking when he says, "Yes star. Yes ster. Pester. Wadda you want. Yes, please. I want um. It's bad. Yes, come on. Mester ander ander ee. I can use um oh my gosh yes!"

There's someone in there, but who?

He talks to everyone. The little red bird ornament on our Christmas tree turns out to be quite a conversationalist.

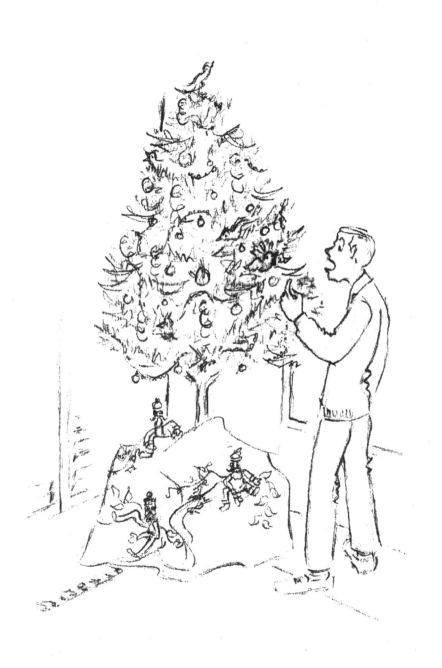

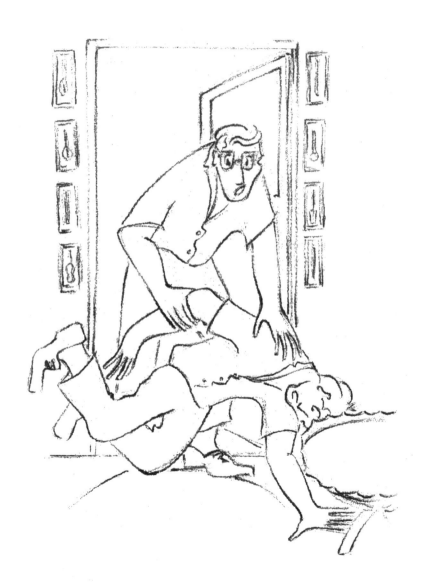

Eighth Year New Year's Eve, Sun City

Coming in from a late after-dinner walk on New Year's Eve, Hank loses his footing. He hits his head on the edge of our brass tray. Paul is completely unnerved. Blood is everywhere. I try to keep calm enough to tend to Hank.

Having brought up three kids, I fervently hope this is more "gore than sore." It isn't. It requires a trip to the Emergency Room and eight stitches. What a way to welcome the New Year!

How will this wound heal? Will Hank worry it all the time? Miraculously, he seems to forget it once he's stitched.

Points to Remember

1. *AD patients will wander. Vigilance is essential.*
2. *Check public systems for finding and returning wanderers.*
3. *Accept help from police and strangers.*
4. *Include grandchildren in family security plans.*
5. *Include AD grandparents in regular family fun.*
6. *A complete break from routine greatly aids caregiver survival.*
7. *Buy easy-on, easy-off clothing.*
8. *Wait out patient's moods. Arguing will not help.*
9. *Expect regression to "second childhood."*
10. *Try to maintain as normal a life as you can for as long as possible.*

V

Coping Day to Day

THE NINTH YEAR

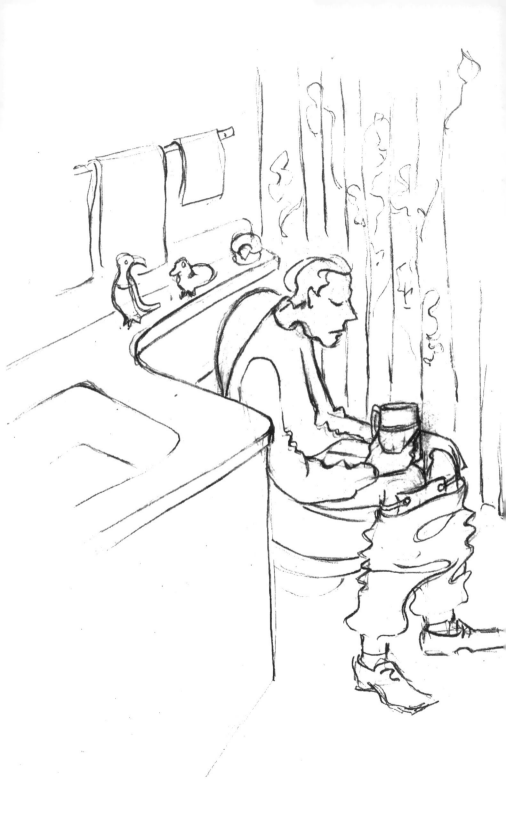

Ninth Year Winter, Sun City West

Answering Hank's calls of nature is one of our primary activities, although we almost never seem to get the timing right.

When they come back from one of their long treks, Paul enthrones Hank, puts a beer in his hand, and hopes the whole ambiance will inspire Hank to tend to business and not just doze off.

I try to keep protective covers on any furniture where Hank might sit, but my success rate is almost nil.

Wall-to-wall carpeting can be a liability as well. I take up every rug I've got. At least THOSE can be rolled away from harm.

I am often so exhausted I wonder if I can get up mornings, but I know I must. I try to sneak out early, before Hank wakes, to walk or ride my bike. I endeavor to get an hour of brisk aerobics at least a couple of times a week.

In bad weather I can keep in shape by doing calisthenics along with one of the TV exercise gurus, using a tape, or peddling an exercise bike.

Keeping in shape is a cheap health insurance policy. Hank can't take over if I get sick.

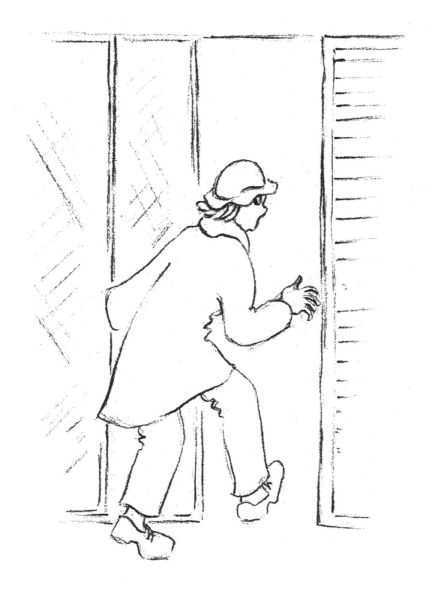

Keeping up with at least a few outside activities becomes increasingly important to me. When and if I can get away, I look forward to a once-a-week bridge game and lectures at our little Sun Cities Art Museum.

A shopping trip, a movie, or a luncheon out with friends works wonders for the psyche. And in summer after a sail or a swim, I always feel refreshed and able to face things better when I get home.

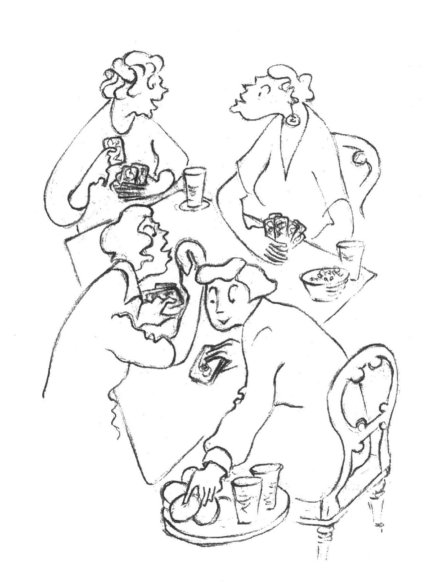

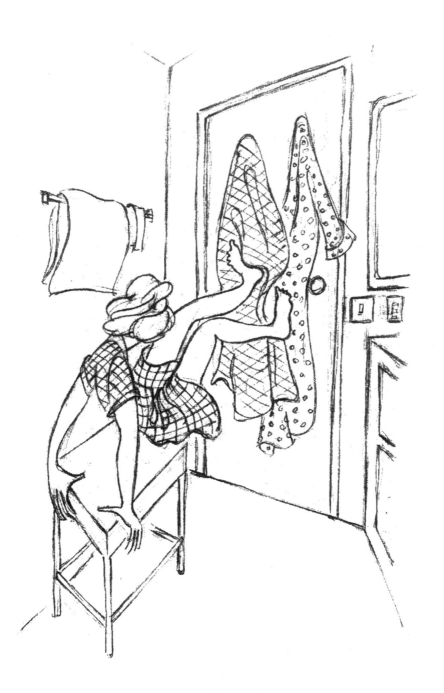

Often I wake up about 3 a.m. with a scary feeling. That's the hour when demons seem to catch up with Hank. For a small man, he is unusually strong. When I sense his violence mounting, I know I must avoid his vise-like grip.

I barricade myself in the bathroom and let Hank rant on, hoping the mood will soon pass. I realize that Paul is within calling distance if things start getting out of hand.

So far Hank's medication has been minimal. We don't want to over medicate, but now Hank's doctor tells us, "Increase the dosage slightly for a while."

Things improve.

Changing positions from standing to sitting gets difficult. At the same time, Hank develops a decided right-hand list. I'm afraid he may fall.

Hank is so often off-balance, we don't dare take him for outdoor walks anymore. Still, he's always in motion. Around and around the house he goes.

With his fists clenched, his face tense and anguished, his breathing heavy, he'll say in desperation, "Let's go! Come on, let's go!"

His hands will often shake nervously. Is he doing this voluntarily? Is Alzheimer's related to Parkinson's?

It's disconcerting when I can't understand what's distressing him. If only I knew what he wanted, I might be able to help.

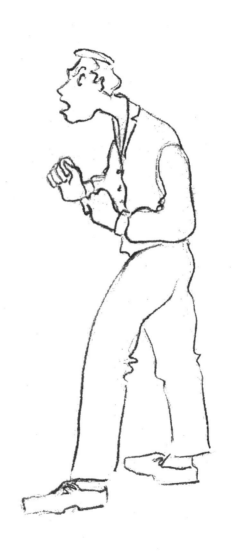

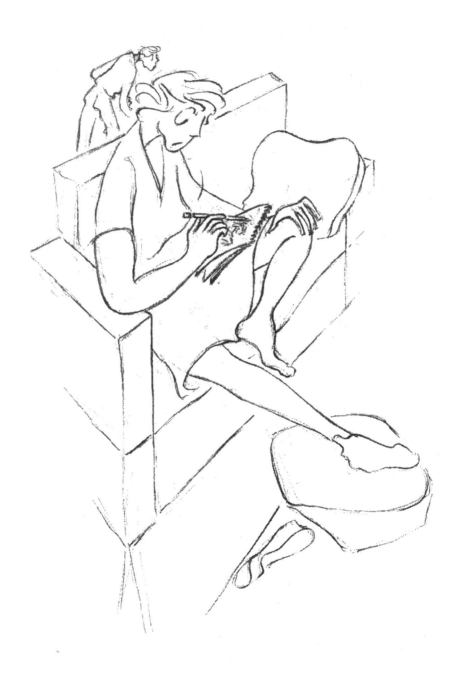

More and more friends retreat. Social invitations slow to a trickle. Instead of acting natural, most people seem not to know how to handle the situation, how to react, what to say, seem to feel embarrassed. Even Hank's brothers are uncomfortable. One is broken up with emotion. The other prefers to ignore the whole thing.

Whereas Paul and I used to take Hank with us most everywhere we went, it's no longer possible. As long as Hank is fed, watered, kept clean, he gets on fine. Now, while Hank shuffles around the house, Paul and I concentrate on our own "home" work. It's getting to be a lonely, isolated life.

I've put aside
the hopes we had
the dreams we shared.
Now I have to think instead
of how to cope alone
with each new day ahead.

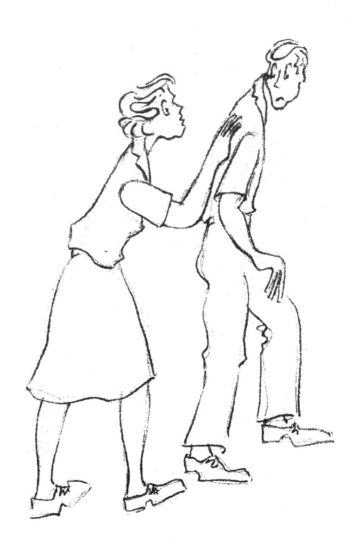

Hank's changed a lot recently. If I need to propel him to a specific location, I have to steer him surely, slowly and gently. He doesn't like to be hurried or pushed.

It shocks me to realize I've begun to think of Hank quite impersonally: as a patient, someone who needs to be cared for. I now avoid looking directly at his face or making eye contact. I couldn't cope if I kept seeing him as he used to be.

The Bible has always been very important to Hank. During his working years, he would get up several hours before he had to leave for work to read and study. Sunday was his "special day," with Church a first priority.

Now, with his span of attention so short, he keeps wanting to get up during the service and go home. His balance is questionable, taking communion is awkward for him. The minister is understanding and considerate, but Hank seems neither to comprehend anything nor care.

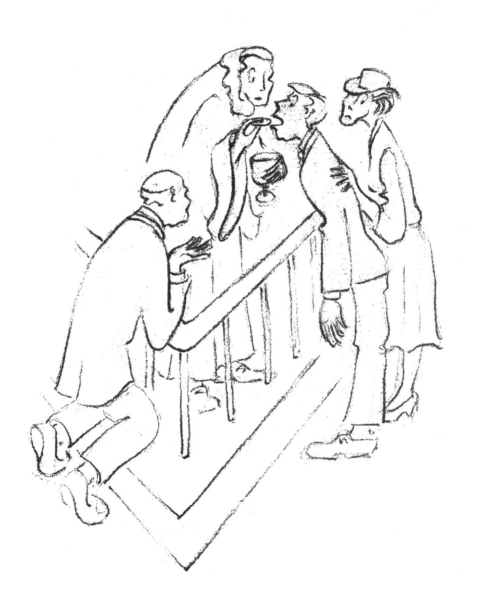

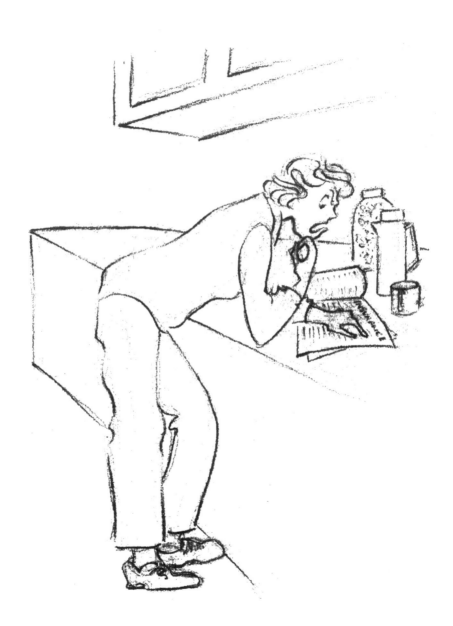

Ninth Year Spring, Sun City West

I'm beginning to wonder how long I can hang on. When I read over the long-term care insurance policy we took out before Hank was diagnosed, I'm shocked to realize it doesn't cover Alzheimer's! My insurance man assures me he explained this thoroughly. Maybe I wasn't listening. New policies, he tells me, are much more comprehensive.

Obviously I need to do some planning for both our futures. How long CAN I keep him home? Waiting lists can be long, so if and when a nursing home is necessary, where will he go? What will the costs be? Can I cover the expenses? How will I organize my life without him?

So many questions to be answered. So many decisions to be made.

As an artist and clothing designer, my activities have been greatly curtailed. But now I have an order for some of my hand-printed originals. These sweat shirts have to be delivered before we leave for Cape Cod.

After three hours of nonstop printing, the last shirt is finally done. Now comes the crucial step, to get the last shirt hung on the line without smudging the wet ink.

I'm called to the phone.

Horrors! When I return, I see Hank has tramped over everything, leaving big, black shoe prints in his wake. I could KILL him!

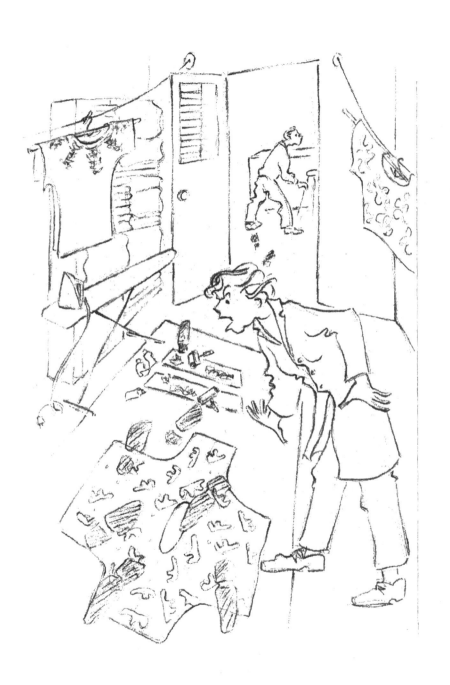

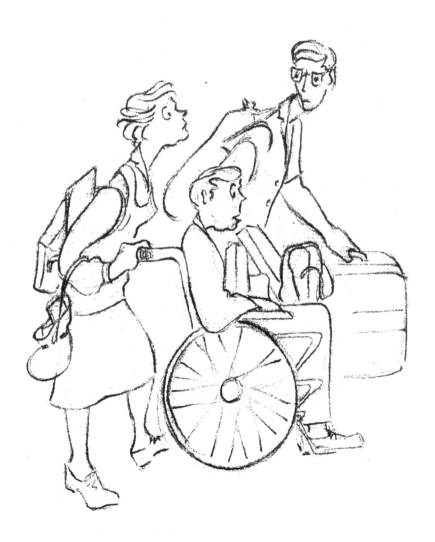

Ninth Year Spring, En Route

Though Hank CAN walk, he's slow. A wheelchair provided by the airline helps us avoid the chance of missing a connecting flight. It makes our hand luggage lighter, too. Compared to previous air trips, we three have finally gotten our act together. We're the epitome of travel efficiency.

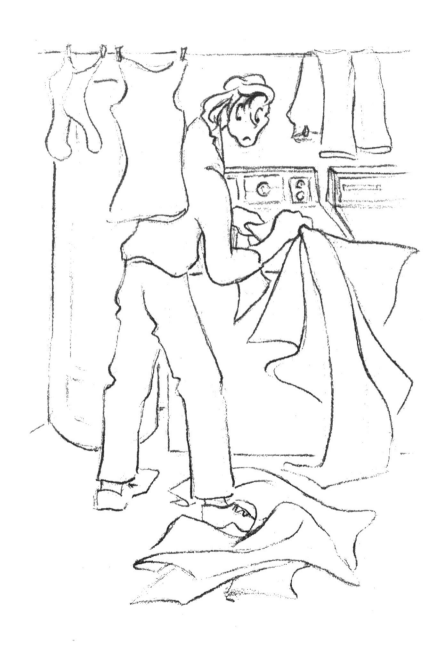

Ninth Year Spring, Cape Cod

Laundry is never ending and mountainous. If I get through a day without a load or two, I think I'm lucky. Hank generates more laundry than one-year-old twins.

Wet bottoms are something I thought I'd left behind with babies. But this "baby" is an adult and won't outgrow his condition. No protection I can find will keep him dry through a whole day or night.

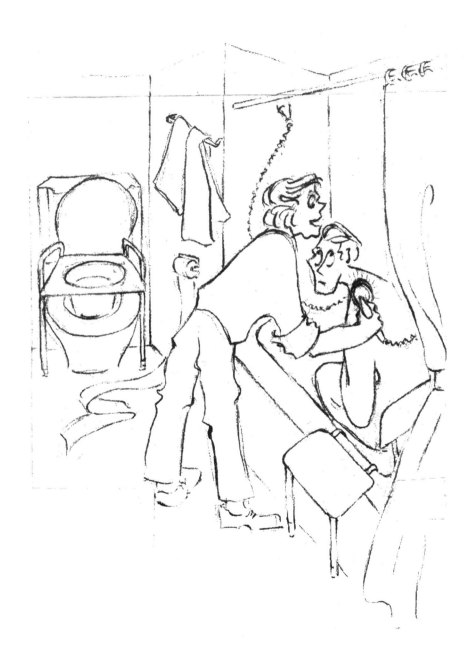

It's like discovering America for me to find products that can simplify the daily "necessaries." At a friend's suggestion we raise the toilet seat, put a cross-over seat in the tub and install a hand-held shower.

I'm so awkward with the shower, I end up even wetter than Hank, and with a flooded floor. Are these gadgets really helpful after all?

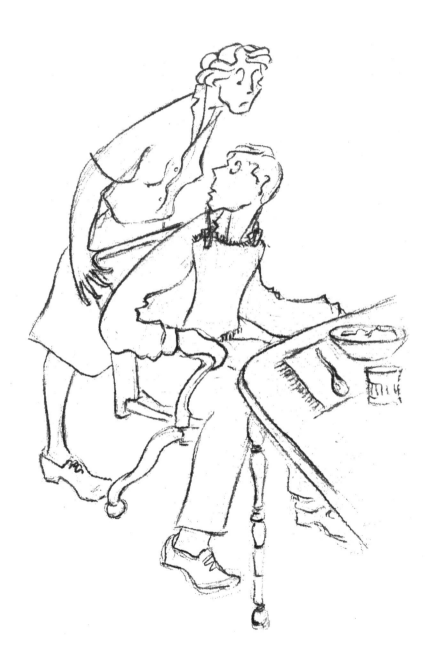

E ating gets more and more complicated. To get Hank closer to the table easily, Paul confiscates my favorite swivel desk chair.

Things improve further when we substitute bowls for plates, spoons for forks, make a bib holder out of a couple of clothes pins and some string.

Hank can be exasperating. He will feed himself until the edge is off his appetite, he loses interest, or just forgets what he's doing. Then we have to feed him. But he ALWAYS comes alive if ice cream is on the menu.

I thought messy mealtimes were over when our kids passed toddlerhood.

How wrong can you be?

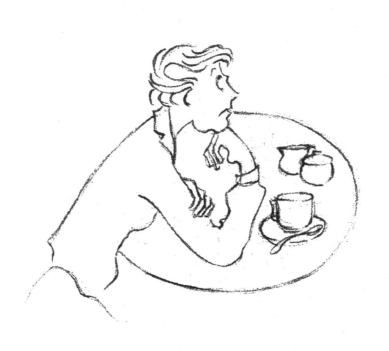

Ninth Year Summer, Cape Cod

Someone always needs to be in attendance, but as long as we give Hank TLC, he's content. It would be harder, I think, to care for someone whose body fails and whose mind is clear.

As my friend, Brownie, says, "If we put everyone's troubles in a hat, and had to choose one, we'd probably choose our own."

Alzheimer's has become far more widely known than when Hank was first diagnosed. Now when anyone forgets, wanders off, or does something bizarre, people often guess (seriously or in jest), "It must be Alzheimer's." In reality, it could be anything from normal aging to a mild stroke, or over medication.

"How do you KNOW it's Alzheimer's?" I'm asked repeatedly. "Doctors tell me that tests by qualified professionals are the only way to come up with a reasonable diagnosis."

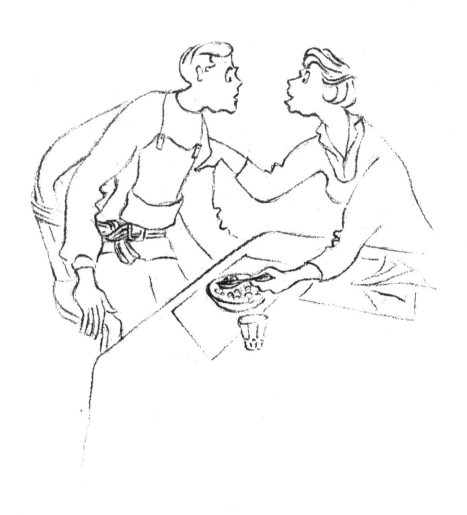

Hank gets more and more unsteady. Some days he can't seem to stay upright at all. Elastic belts keep him comfortably attached to the swivel chair. We don't want him to be completely immobilized, of course, so we keep getting him up to test his balance. Often he can stand and walk safely as the day wears on, sometimes not.

The belts work wonders, too, when on his steady days Hank pops up after each bite he's fed. Mealtimes would be endless were he allowed to roam at will.

For a few months Hank's balance returns to normal. Is he in remission? Is it safe to take him on walks again? He has good and bad days.

Then, many evenings he goes limp. He has little control when he sits. He's reluctant, or unable, to help himself rise.

I don't look forward to getting him ready for bed. Sometimes I have, literally, to lift him to his feet.

Paul's generally "off duty" at night, but at least he's within calling distance if I need him.

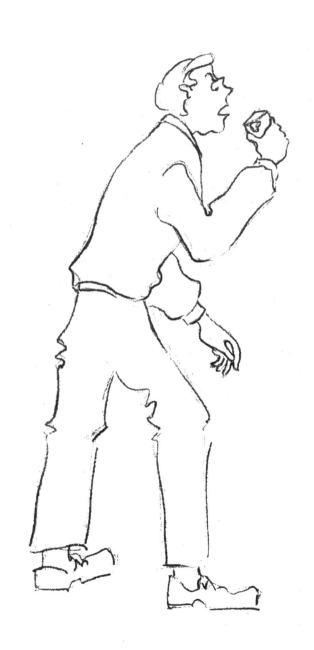

Hank refuses to brush his teeth anymore. It's all but impossible to do it for him. Then I remember our dentist once said, "If you can't brush, eat fruit or raw vegetables."

We leave apple slices, celery and carrot sticks where Hank can get them easily as he passes, plying him with them in between meals.

After finishing off all the cut-up fruit and vegetables Paul has left for him to munch, Hank looks for something more.

The yellow bar of laundry soap looks very appealing . . . until he takes a bite.

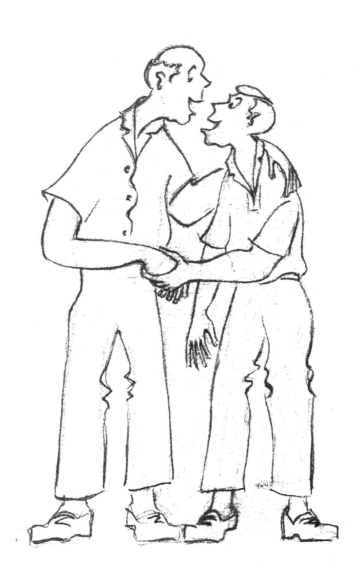

There ARE some friends with whom we still feel comfortable and who feel comfortable with us. When we go for drinks, Hank's greeted with, "Well, old buddy, how are you tonight?"

Hank smiles broadly and clasps his friend's hand. Though most of his other speech is garbled, he surprises us by saying clearly, "Yes. Yes. I love you. Yes I do."

Is there a glimmer of recognition?

My eye isn't firmly focused on Hank when I'm out planting tomatoes. Asher looks up from his crabbing just in time to spot Hank wandering off into the woods. He scurries to the rescue, takes Hank's hand and says, "Come on, Grandpa, this way," and leads Hank gently home.

Grandsons, charged with 100-volt batteries, may be utterly exhausting, but they are lovely little people, too.

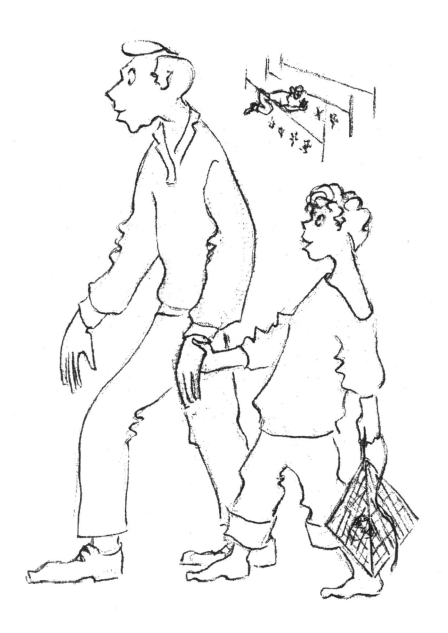

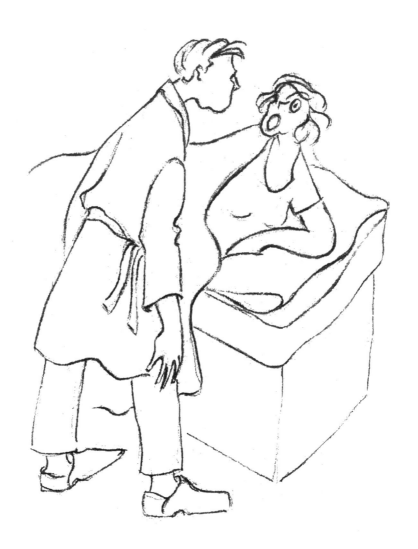

Ninth Year Fall, Cape Cod

After changing Hank and his sheets at about midnight, I try to lead him back to bed. He won't have any of it. He will only let me help him into MY bathrobe and HIS slippers.

Knowing I can get nowhere until he calms down, I decide to doze with one eye open.

Next thing I know it's morning! I'm horrified to realize Hank's been roaming around the room for over six hours! I'm glad it's early September instead of January. How can I be so neglectful and thoughtless?

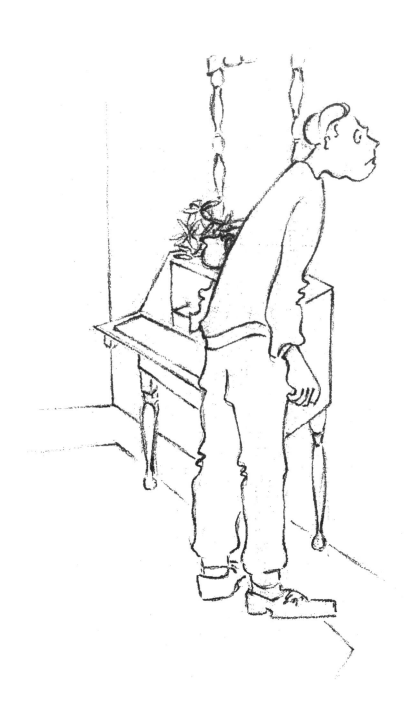

P aul's elaborate security system has become obsolete. Things are a bit easier now since Hank hardly ever wanders away. He will no longer even try to open any closed door or gate.

When Hank interrupts his pacing, he comes to rest, facing a blank wall. It seems to mesmerize him. It's as if, having hit a barrier, he can't quite figure out how to get around or through it.

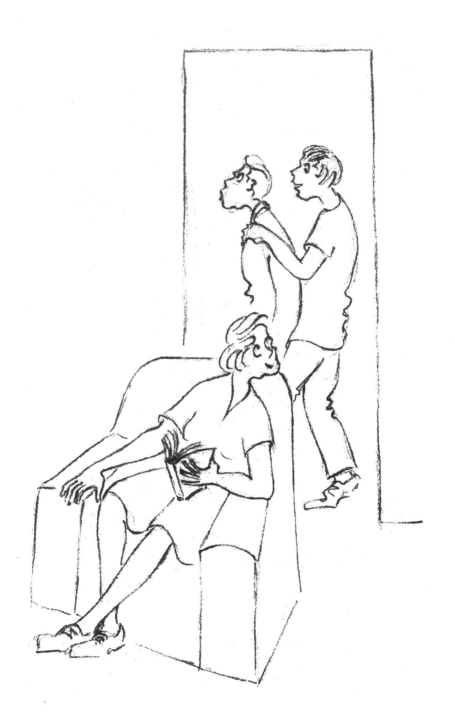

During family visits, it's wonderful to have an occasional respite from the daily routine. Still, I can't help feeling a little guilty when Tuck or one of the girls gets Hank ready for bed, or does some other necessary chore for him. It's MY responsibility, after all. I shouldn't lay that on them when they're so busy and here for such a short time.

"You're wrong, Mom," they tell me. "We want to help Dad. It makes us feel more a part of what's going on and to understand a little of what you're going through. Don't shut us out."

I've been so engrossed in doing MY job, I've never even considered how THEY might feel.

The entire family gathers for Kate and Terry's wedding. The big day arrives. The sun comes out from behind rain clouds just fifteen minutes before the outdoor ceremony is to begin.

I'm amazed at the people (close family as well as casual friends) who ask, "What will you do with Hank during the wedding?"

Why do they wonder? He's the bride's father, isn't he? OF COURSE he'll be there! Kate and Terry wouldn't have it any other way.

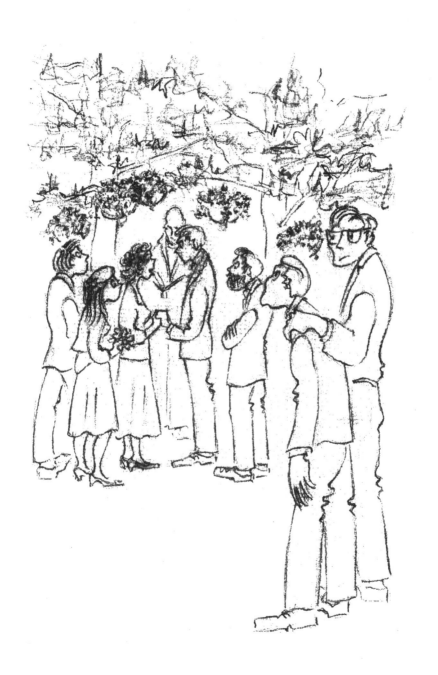

In late September Paul does the honors while I'm off on a shopping spree. Returning at 3 p.m., I find the place in an uproar. Firemen, medics, police are everywhere. The rancid smell of smoke permeates everything.

We've been burned out of our house! I'm in shock!

Where's Hank? No one seems to know. I should have guessed. He's safe and sound, penned in the garage. Paul has him snugly wrapped in an old, dirty, derelict quilt resurrected from heaven knows where.

How did this get started? The fire chief explains that the culprit is the fireplace fire Paul has been making daily to cheer and warm us. A minute, hidden flue fault allowed the flames to escape up through the living room wall. The whole middle of the house has been gutted.

We'll have to stay in rented quarters until we go back to Arizona. Arrangements must be made to repair the house. It will be longer than I'd wish before we can go back to Sun City West. Why does this have to happen to us?

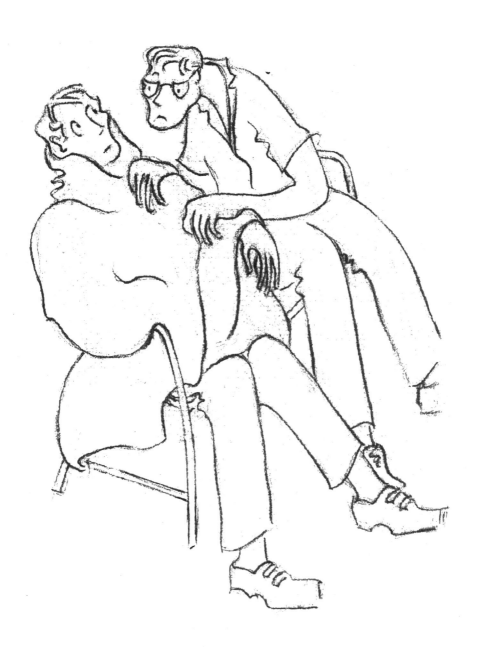

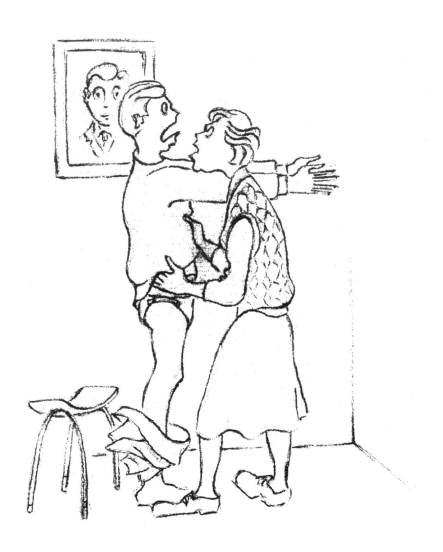

It's the day after Thanksgiving. Everything appears normal as I begin to get Hank ready for the day.

Suddenly, he lets out a bloodcurdling scream. His body becomes rigid. His face is ashen. He falls to the floor in a faint. Fortunately, I'm able to grab him in time to break his descent so that he doesn't crash and hurt himself. He's swallowing so much phlegm I'm afraid he may choke. I'm nearly fainting myself.

Mary, my sister who is here for the holiday, takes control, tells me to call for help . . .

Again the town emergency services rush to our rescue. With me in the front seat and siren screeching, the ambulance speeds us to the hospital. Once there, the doctor assures me nothing is additionally wrong. He tells me that Alzheimer's victims often suffer seizures, and that if it happens again, I should remember to turn Hank on his side.

Back home, I realize I need not have panicked. I hope I can handle things better next time.

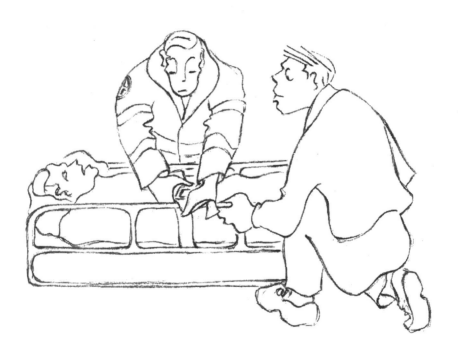

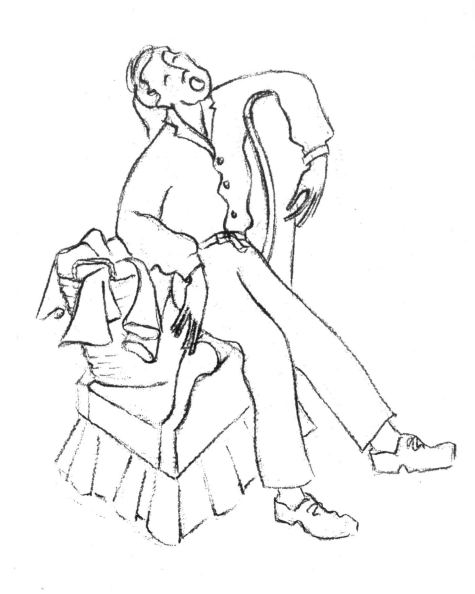

I hear a loud snore. There's Hank, asleep anywhere, on most anything. He does this frequently now.

> *GONE?*
> *ears hear*
> *nose smells*
> *tongue tastes*
> *fingers feel*
> *eyes see*
> *there may even be*
> *ESP*
> *but who can answer*
> *"Where is he?"*

Points to Remember

1. Protect furniture and rugs, as if a baby were in the house.
2. Keep up outside interests and activities.
3. To minimize AD mood swings and possible violent behavior, consult a doctor for medication.
4. Coping is easier if patient is treated impersonally.
5. Be aware that patient's attendance at church services and social gatherings will become unacceptable to others.
6. Consider the use of a wheelchair.
7. Install bathroom aids for easier care.
8. Simplify mealtimes with swivel chair, bib, spoon and a bowl.
9. Devise a comfortable seatbelt to avoid meal-time wandering.
10. When tooth brushing fails, offer carrots, apple slices.
11. Include family members in patient care.
12. Learn first aid for seizures, which are aptt to occur.

VI

The Curtain Closes

THE TENTH YEAR

Tenth Year Summer, Cape Cod

Neither Paul nor I can understand why Hank begins to lift his feet off the floor when he sits, and why he is suddenly reluctant to walk even when we hold him.

Paul finally realizes Hank has developed large blisters on both heels. One blister is broken and bloody. We think his shoes are to blame. But we can't chance infection.

Getting Hank to the Doctor's office presents a new problem. With his feet too sore to walk on, he must be carried. He seems to weigh a ton.

Linda, the office nurse, hasn't seen Hank in a long time. She's appalled at how far downhill he's gone.

Paul and I have been so close to Hank for so long we've hardly noticed. Through Linda's eyes we see how frail and disabled he really is.

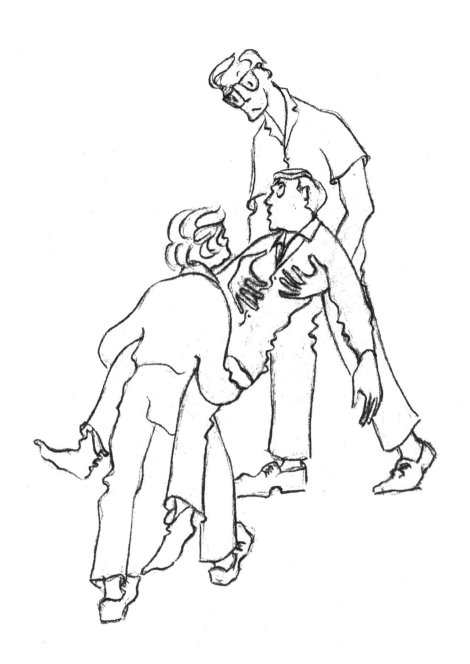

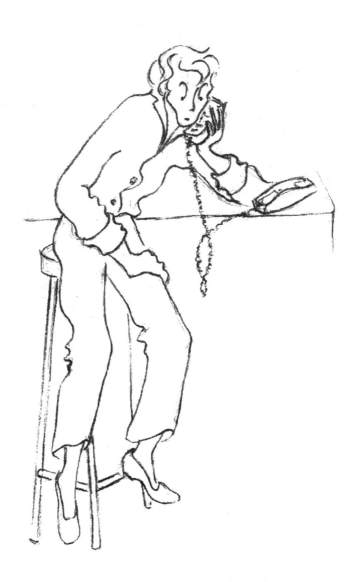

D r. Burwell tells us these heel blisters, resulting from blanket pressure, can be cured by using padded booties and keeping Hank off his feet until they heal.

Is it possible that Hank will be completely immobile from now on? I haven't wanted to think of this. Sadly, I arrange for a wheelchair. Next I look into Dr. Burwell's other recommendations: respite care, where professionals can supervise things in a controlled environment, and/or the help of a visiting nurse who can advise on the best care for a bedridden Hank at home. Perhaps we can hold on a little longer.

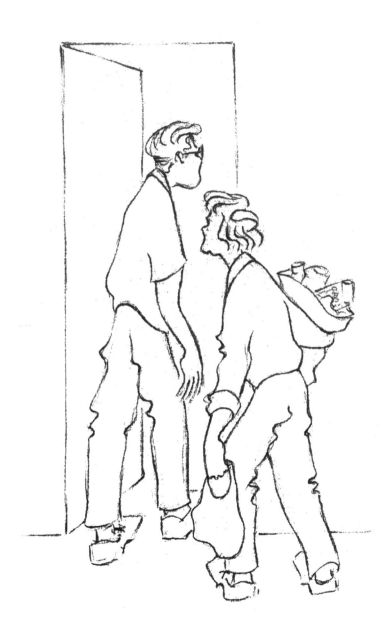

After doing some early morning shopping I return home to a soundless house. Silently Paul leads me into the bedroom . . .

No need for a wheelchair . . .

No need for a visiting nurse . . .

No need for respite care . . .

My Hank is gone.

Cardiac arrest is the doctor's official pronouncement. "How can that be?" I ask. "Was not Alzheimer's even remotely responsible?"

"Not ultimately," I'm told.

Except as a statistic, it really doesn't matter, I suppose.

Surely, it doesn't ease the pain.

Paul and I should have been prepared for Hank's death. But how can anyone be? Suddenly, my life is empty, without focus. For ten long years Hank has been the center of all my thoughts and activities. His illness has controlled every waking and sleeping hour.

I feel guilty, but it's a relief to have the burden lifted. Over and over I tell myself, "Hank and I are free again."

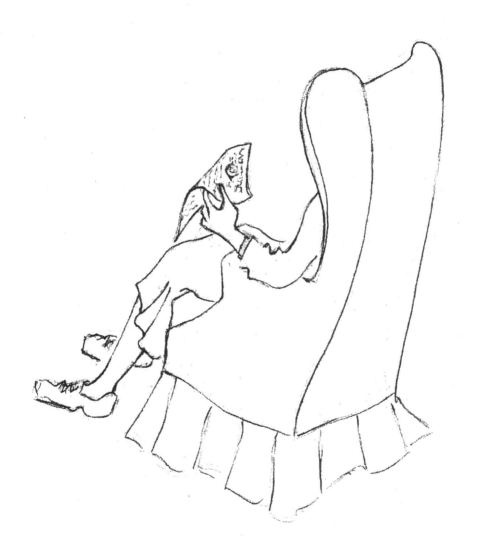

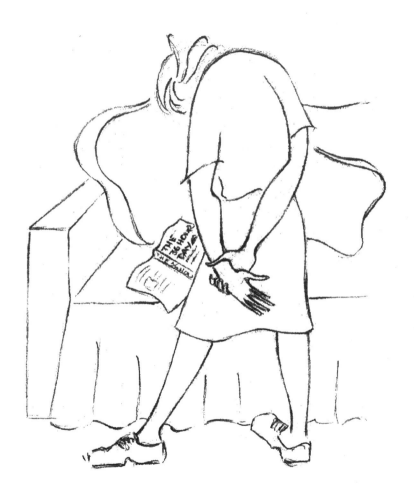

Epilogue

I wish I could mourn, but I can't even cry. I'm numb. The light that was Hank went out a very long time ago. Now I want only to remember the Hank I once knew . . .

the Hank who spent five years under the Pacific as a submariner during World War II and was mustered out as a Lieutenant Commander . . .

the Hank who was one of the youngest overseas operations managers his company ever appointed; who built and managed oil terminals with hundreds of men under his direction and was honored for his work; who refused promotions with more power and position because he knew what he liked to do . . .

the Hank who loved gardenias and roses, planting gardens of them wherever we lived, tending them with TLC . . .

the Hank who spent hours patiently training each one of our five assorted mongrels . . .

the Hank who was keeper of sixty-four beehives and once helped firemen extricate a bee swarm from a traffic light on a main boulevard . . .

the Hank who jogged ten miles a day years before
jogging was the "in" thing to do . . .

the Hank who, as a married man, thought he should
learn to drink coffee and play cards, never mastering
either . . .

who cradled our sick baby all night as I slept . . .

who was a lay reader and for whom the Bible was
a way of life . . .

the Hank who worked steadily on his finances
throughout his career so that we would be indepen-
dent in retirement . . .

who, with one helper, built our first little house
on Cape Cod with enough land for a lifetime of
tending, then planted hundreds of evergreen
seedlings, and loved every one of them . . .

the Hank who always championed the underdog,
but could not tolerate a loafer . . .

the Hank who always said that what he lacked in
brains he made up for in hard work . . .

who made all the decisions . . .

paid all the bills . . .

was on top of everything.

I loved that Hank

I will miss him . . . always.

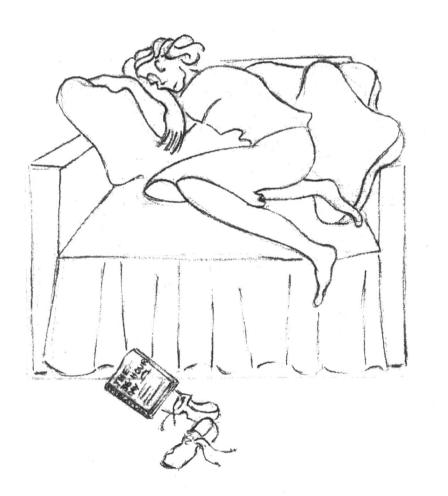

BETTY BAKER SPOHR

After graduating from Skidmore College with a fine arts degree, Betty Baker worked in freelance card and package designing, mannequin making and retail window design in New York City, and New Jersey where she grew up. With the Red Cross during World War II, she helped run recreational clubs for enlisted men in Africa, Sicily, and Italy. Returning to the States, she worked in New York City as a fashion copy writer.

Her marriage to engineer Hank Spohr took her to Indonesia, Vietnam, Kenya, South Africa and Nigeria. Betty sketched continually during her overseas years and perfected her skills in fashion design and block printing. Three children and twenty-five years later, the Spohrs returned to retire in the States. At retirement, Betty received the shattering diagnosis of Hank's Alzheimer's disease.

Catch a Falling Star is Betty's story of ten years spent coping with and caring for Hank at home. Now Betty Baker Spohr divides her time between Sun City West, Arizona, and Cape Cod, Massachusetts.

JEAN VALENS BULLARD

Catch a Falling Star was created and developed with the assistance and guidance of editor, author, and freelance writer Jean Valens Bullard. Jean is a Mount Holyoke College graduate and former publications specialist with the National Park Service. She, and her park naturalist husband Bill, raised four children while employed in national parks. They currently live in Seattle, Washington, where they enjoy the Pacific Northwest. An active member of Outdoor Writers Association of America, Jean continues to write about parks, camping, hiking, skiing, and world travel.

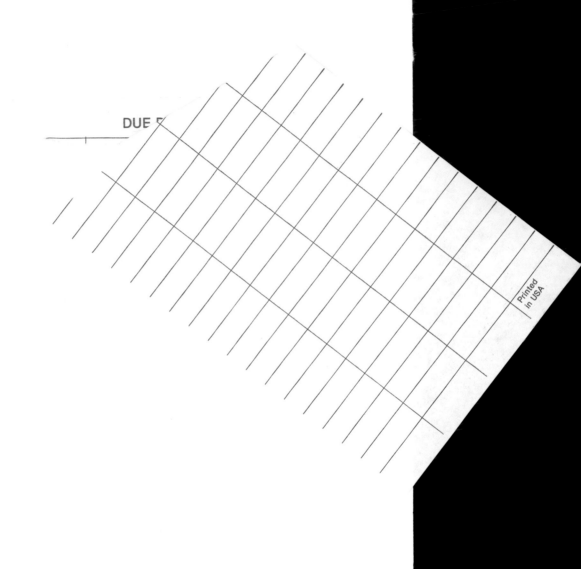

DUE

Printed in USA